Step by Step
Phacoemulsification

System requirements:

- Operating System—Windows Vista or above
- Web Browser—Google Chrome, Mozilla Firefox, Internet Explorer 9 and above
- Essential plugins—Java and Flash player
  - Facing problems in viewing content—it may be your system does not have Java enabled.
  - If videos do not show up—it may be the system requires Flash player or need to manage flash setting. To learn more about Flash setting, click on the link in the help section.
  - You can test Java and Flash by using the links from the help section of the CD/DVD.

Accompanying DVD-ROM is playable only in Computer and not in DVD player.
CD/DVD has autorun function—it may take few seconds to load on your computer. If it does not work for you, then follow the steps below to access the contents manually:

- Click on my computer
- Select the **CD/DVD** drive and click open/explore—this will show list of files in the **CD/DVD**
- Find and double click file—"launch.html"

For more information about troubleshoot of Autorun click on: (http://support.microsoft.com/kb/330135)

DVD Contents

1. Angle Kappa and Multifocal Glued IOL
2. Intraocular Lens (IOL) Scaffold
3. Lens Coloboma
4. Mature Cataract + Adherent Leucoma + Posterior Synechia
5. No-assistant Technique
6. Pars Plicata Anterior Vitrectomy (PPAV)
7. Subluxated Bag—IOL Complex with Dislocated Ring and Endocapsular Segment

Step by Step® **Phacoemulsification**

Third Edition

Editors

Amar Agarwal MS FRCS FRCOphth

Chairman and Managing Director
Dr Agarwal's Group of Eye Hospitals and Eye Research Center
Chennai, Tamil Nadu, India

Priya Narang MS

Director
Narang Eye Care and Laser Center
Ahmedabad, Gujarat, India

Foreword
Audrey Talley Rostov

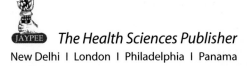

The Health Sciences Publisher
New Delhi I London I Philadelphia I Panama

Jaypee Brothers Medical Publishers (P) Ltd.

Headquarters

Jaypee Brothers Medical Publishers (P) Ltd.
4838/24, Ansari Road, Daryaganj
New Delhi 110 002, India
Phone: +91-11-43574357
Fax: +91-11-43574314
Email: jaypee@jaypeebrothers.com

Overseas Offices

J.P. Medical Ltd.
83, Victoria Street, London
SW1H 0HW (UK)
Phone: +44 20 3170 8910
Fax: +44 (0)20 3008 6180
Email: info@jpmedpub.com

Jaypee-Highlights Medical Publishers Inc.
City of Knowledge, Bld. 237, Clayton
Panama City, Panama
Phone: +1 507-301-0496
Fax: +1 507-301-0499
Email: cservice@jphmedical.com

Jaypee Medical Inc.
The Bourse
111, South Independence Mall East
Suite 835, Philadelphia
PA 19106, USA
Phone: +1 267-519-9789
Email: jpmed.us@gmail.com

Jaypee Brothers Medical Publishers (P) Ltd.
17/1-B, Babar Road, Block-B
Shaymali, Mohammadpur
Dhaka-1207, Bangladesh
Mobile: +08801912003485
Email: jaypeedhaka@gmail.com

Jaypee Brothers Medical Publishers (P) Ltd.
Bhotahity, Kathmandu, Nepal
Phone: +977-9741283608
Email: kathmandu@jaypeebrothers.com

Website: www.jaypeebrothers.com
Website: www.jaypeedigital.com

© 2015, Jaypee Brothers Medical Publishers

Step by Step® Phacoemulsification

First Edition: 2005
Second Edition: 2006
Third Edition: **2015**
ISBN: 978-93-5152-783-1
Printed at : Samrat Offset Pvt. Ltd.

Dedicated to

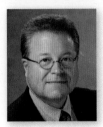

Warren Hill

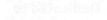

Contributors

Amar Agarwal MS FRCS FRCOphth
Chairman and Managing Director
Dr Agarwal's Group of Eye Hospitals and
Eye Research Center
Chennai, Tamil Nadu, India

Ashvin Agarwal MS
Director
Dr Agarwal's Group of Eye Hospital and
Eye Research Center
Chennai, Tamil Nadu, India

Clement K Chan MD FACS
Medical Director
Southern California Desert
Retina Consultants, Medical Center
Inland Retina Consultants
Palm Springs, California, USA

Associate Clinical Professor
Department of Ophthalmology
Loma Linda University
Loma Linda, California, USA

Priya Narang MS
Director
Narang Eye Care and Laser Center
Ahmedabad, Gujarat, India

Steven G Lin MD
Southern California Desert
Retina Consultants, Medical Center
Inland Retina Consultants
Palm Springs, California, USA

Contributors

Foreword to the Third Edition

Cataract is a significant global health problem and a leading cause of blindness worldwide. Although great strides have been made in the field of cataract and anterior segment surgery, there is still much work to be done. Since the introduction of phacoemulsification by Dr Charles Kelman over 40 years ago, there have been significant surgical advancements in phaco technology and IOL techniques.

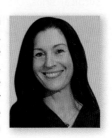

Dr Amar Agarwal and his colleagues are innovators in the field of cataract and anterior segment surgery and are especially well known for their popularization of glued IOL techniques. They have a wealth of experience in complex case scenarios and are internationally applauded for their informative presentations on transforming the "Longest Day" in the operating suite into sight-restoring cataract surgical procedures.

With the third edition of *Step by Step® Phacoemulsification*, Drs Amar Agarwal and Priya Narang deliver another compilation of cataract surgical techniques designed to teach both the comprehensive cataract surgeons as well as the advanced anterior segment reconstructive surgeons. This step-by-step textbook provides a matrix for surgical decision making and learning a variety of cataract surgical techniques as well as the management of intraoperative and postoperative complications. Well-researched and beautifully illustrated topics include the management of mature cataracts, subluxated cataracts and endocapsular ring segments, small pupil phaco, phakonit and microphakonit, glued IOL and IOL scaffold techniques and the management of infectious endophthalmitis and cystoid macular edema.

The authors demonstrate a commitment to continuous improvement in patient care by providing strands of phaco pearls obtained from their vast clinical and surgical experiences. Through the advancement of education and teaching of cataract surgical skills, Drs Agarwal and colleagues provide us with this comprehensive approach to help eliminate blindness and restore vision from this very treatable disease.

Audrey Talley Rostov MD
Cornea, Cataract and
Refractive Surgeon

Foreword to the Second Edition

The topic of this book needs no introduction. Cataract surgery has been at the forefront of ophthalmic consciousness forever. Cataract, opacification of the lens, is one of the most common causes of loss of useful vision, with an estimated 16 million people worldwide affected. Several risk factors have been identified in addition to increasing age 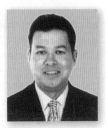 including genetic composition, exposure to ultraviolet light, and diabetes. However, no method to halt the formation of a cataractous lens has been shown to be effective. Nevertheless, advances in surgical removal of cataracts, including small-incision surgery, use of viscoelastics, and the development of intraocular lenses, have made treatment very effective and visual recovery rapid in most cases. Despite these advances, cataract continues to be a leading public-health issue that will grow in importance as the population increases and life expectancy is extended worldwide.

Phacoemulsification, first developed by Kelman in 1967, is currently the procedure of choice for the surgical management of cataracts. The search continues for innovations that allow easier manipulation of intraocular lenses through even smaller incisions. The smaller incision in phacoemulsification allows for the maintenance of a near-normal anterior chamber during surgery, decreasing the risks. Smaller incisions have decreased the duration of the procedure and, more importantly, hastened postoperative visual recovery. Dr Amar Agarwal and colleagues have become one of the most important modern-day innovators with the invention of revolutionary techniques such as phakonit. Cataract removal through a sub-1.0 mm incision and implantation of a rollable intraocular lens, and no-anesthesia clear corneal phacoemulsification.

For these reasons, the appearance of the second edition of *Dr Agarwals' Step by Step Series on Phaco* by Drs Sunita Agarwal, Athiya Agarwal, and Amar Agarwal to help ophthalmologists learn the newest techniques on cataract surgery is a wonderful gift to all of us and our patients. The book has been beautifully illustrated and divided into 12 masterful chapters including important topics such as Gas Forced Infusion, No Anesthesia Cataract Surgery with the Karate Chop Technique, Phaco in Subluxated Cataracts, Mature Cataracts, Small Pupil Phacoemulsification, Combined Cataract and Glaucoma Surgery, Managing Dislocated Lens Fragments, The Malpositioned Intraocular Implant, Infectious Endophthalmitis, Cystoid Macular Edema, *Bimanual Phaco/Phakonit/MICS*: Surgical Technique, *Microphakonit*: Cataract Surgery with A 0.7 mm Tip.

Contributors of this book are both educators and treaters. There was no way for them to have developed these techniques except to do it. Their accumulated knowledge is the result of tremendous clinical and academic efforts and their expertise flows to the reader with the hope that individual lives will benefit. In bringing their work to press, Drs Sunita Agarwal, Athiya Agarwal, and Amar Agarwal have done a great service to patients living with cataracts and to the doctors caring for them. Those who will read and study this text have already demonstrated that they care for their patients and that they want to learn. We now just need to move forward together to give our patients the gift of sight.

J Fernando Arevalo MD FACS
Clinica Oftalmologica Centro Caracas
The Arevalo-Coutinho Foundation
for Research in Ophthalmology
Caracas, Venezuela

Preface

We are honored to have been asked to edit the third edition of *Step by Step®
Phacoemulsification*. With this edition, we aim to find more knowledgeable and productive information—all in one book. This ambitious goal was set to provide the readers with the most comprehensive and current information covering the broad field within phacoemulsification. It is hoped that the edition captures the current state of the vital and dynamic science from international perspective.

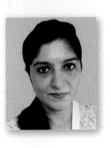

New to the edition are the chapters on handling complications in phacoemulsi-fication surgery areas that have developed significantly in recent years. The remaining chapters have been thoroughly updated to reflect developments since the last edition. The book has a display of chapters on varied topics covering every aspect of phacoemulsification surgery with a brilliant display of figures and videos that have been enrolled in the accompanying interactive DVD-ROM.

We hope that the book will be a valuable reference for readers, health professionals, and a useful resource for educators and established professionals.

Amar Agarwal
Priya Narang

Contents

1

Gas Forced Infusion: Controlling the Surge

Amar Agarwal

HISTORY

The main problem encountered in bimanual phaco/ phakonit was the destabilization of the anterior chamber during surgery. This was solved by us to a certain extent by using an 18-gauge irrigating chopper. Dr Sunita Agarwal suggested the use of an antichamber collapser, which injects air into the infusion bottle (Fig. 1.1). This pushes more fluid into the eye through the irrigating chopper and also prevents surge.[1-11] Thus, we were able to use a 20 gauge or 21 gauge irrigating chopper as well as solve the problem of destabilization of the anterior chamber during surgery. Now with microphakonit and gas forced infusion we are able to remove cataracts with a 0.7 mm irrigating chopper (22 gauge). Subsequently we used this system in all our co-axial phaco cases including microincisional co-axial phaco to prevent complications like posterior capsular ruptures and corneal damage.

INTRODUCTION

Since the introduction of phacoemulsification by Kelman,[1] it has been undergoing revolutionary changes in an attempt to perfect the

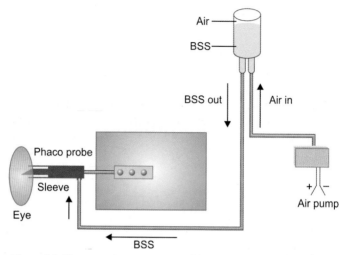

Figure 1.1 Diagrammatic representation of the connection of the air pump to the infusion bottle

techniques of extracapsular cataract extraction surgery. Although advantageous in many aspects, this technique is not without its attending complications. A well maintained anterior chamber without intraocular fluctuations is one of the pre-requisites for safe phacoemulsification and phakonit.[2]

When an occluded fragment is held by high vacuum and then abruptly aspirated, fluid rushes into the phaco tip to equilibrate the built up vacuum in the aspiration line, causing surge.[3] This leads to shallowing or collapse of the anterior chamber. Different machines employ a variety of methods to combat surge. These include usage of noncompliant tubing,[4] small bore aspiration line tubing,[4] microflow tips,[4] aspiration bypass systems,[4] dual linear foot pedal control[4] and incorporation of sophisticated microprocessors[4] to sense the anterior chamber pressure fluctuations.

The surgeon dependent variables to counteract surge include good wound construction with minimal leakage,[5] and selection of appropriate machine parameters depending on the stage of the surgery.[5] An anterior chamber maintainer has also been described in literature to prevent surge, but an extra side port makes it an inconvenient procedure.

We started a simple and effective method to prevent anterior chamber collapse during phacoemulsification and phakonit in 1999 by increasing the velocity of the fluid inflow into the anterior chamber. This is achieved by an automated air pump which pumps atmospheric air through an air filter into the infusion bottle thereby preventing surge. We stumbled upon this idea when we were operating cases with phakonit[7] where we wanted more fluid entering the eye, but even now we use it in all our phacoemulsification cases.[8]

AIR PUMP

An automated air pump is used to push air into the infusion bottle thus increasing the pressure with which the fluid flows into the eye. This increases the steady-state pressure of the eye making the anterior chamber deep and well maintained during the entire procedure. It makes phakonit and phacoemulsification a relatively safe procedure by reducing surge even at high vacuum levels.

TECHNIQUE

A locally manufactured automated device, used in fish tanks (aquariums) to supply oxygen, is utilized to forcefully pump air into the irrigation bottle. This pump is available in aquarium shops and has an electromagnetic motor which moves a lever attached to a collapsible rubber cap. There is an inlet with a valve, which sucks in atmospheric air as the cap expands. On collapsing, the valve closes and the air is pushed into an intravenous (IV) line connected to the infusion bottle (Fig. 1.1). The lever vibrates at a frequency of approximately 10 oscillations per second. The electromagnetic motor is weak enough to stop once the pressure in the closed system (i.e. the anterior chamber) reaches about 50 mm of Hg. The rubber cap ceases to expand at this pressure level. A millipore air filter is used between the air pump and the infusion bottle so that the air pumped into the bottle is clean of the particulate matter.

METHOD

- First of all, the balanced salt solution (BSS) bottle is taken and put on the IV stand.
- Now we take an air pump. This air pump is the kind of air pump, which is used in fish tanks (aquariums) to infuse oxygen to the fishes. The air pump is plugged on to the electrical connection.
- An IV set now connects the air pump to the infusion bottle. The tubing passes from the air pump and the end of the tubing is passed into one of the infusion bottles.
- When the air pump is switched on, it pumps air into the infusion bottle. This air goes to the top of the bottle and because of the pressure; it pumps the fluid down with greater force. With this, the fluid now flows from the infusion bottle to reach the phaco handpiece or irrigating chopper. The amount of fluid now coming out of the hand piece is much more than what would normally come out and with more force.
- A millipore air filter is connected between the air pump and the infusion bottle so that the air which is being pumped into the bottle is sterile.
- This extra amount of fluid coming out compensates for the surge which would otherwise occur.

CONTINUOUS INFUSION

Before we enter the eye, we fill the eye with viscoelastic. Then once the tip of the phaco handpiece in phaco or irrigating chopper in phakonit is inside the anterior chamber we shift to continuous irrigation. This is very helpful especially for surgeons who are in the learning curve of phacoemulsification or phakonit. This way, the surgeon never comes to position zero and the anterior chamber never collapses. Even for excellent surgeons this helps a lot.

ADVANTAGES

- With the air pump, the posterior capsule is pushed back and there is a deep anterior chamber.
- The phenomenon of surge is neutralized. This prevents the unnecessary posterior capsular rupture.
- Striate keratitis postoperatively is reduced, as there is a deep anterior chamber.
- Hard cataracts can be operated quite comfortably, as striate keratitis does not occur postoperatively.
- The surgical time is shorter as one can emulsify the nuclear pieces much faster as surge does not occur.
- One can easily operate cases with the Phakonit technique as quite a lot of fluid now passes into the eye. Thus, the cataract can be removed through a smaller opening.
- It is quite comfortable to do cases under topical or no-anesthesia.

TOPICAL OR NO-ANESTHESIA CATARACT SURGERY

During phacoemulsification under topical or no-anesthesia, the main problem encountered is that sometimes the pressure is high especially if the patient squeezes the eye. In such cases, the posterior capsule comes up anteriorly and one can produce a posterior capsular rupture. To solve this problem, surgeons tend to work more anteriorly, performing supracapsular phacoemulsification/phakonit. The disadvantage of this is that striate keratitis tends to occur.

With the air pump, this problem is solved totally as the posterior capsule is pushed back. In other words, there is a lot of space between the posterior capsule and the cornea, preventing striate keratitis and inadvertent posterior capsular rupture.

INTERNAL GAS FORCED INFUSION

This was started by Arturo Pérez-Arteaga from Mexico. The anterior vented gas forced infusion system (AVGFI) of the accurus surgical system is used.

This is a system incorporated in the Accurus machine that creates a positive infusion pressure inside the eye; it was designed by the Alcon engineers to control the intraocular pressure (IOP) during posterior segment surgery. It consist of an air pump and a regulator which are inside the machine; then the air is pushed inside the bottle of intraocular solution, and so the fluid is actively pushed inside the eye without raising or lowering the bottle. The control of the air pump is digitally integrated in the Accurus panel; it also can be controlled via the remote. Also the footswitch can be preset with the minimal and maximum of desired fluid inside the eye and go directly to this value with the simple touch of the footswitch. Arturo Pérez-Arteaga recommends to preset the infusion pump at 100 mm of Hg; it is enough strong irrigation force to perform a microincision phaco. This parameter is preset in the panel and also as the minimal irrigation force in the footswitch; then he recommends to preset the maximum irrigation force at 130 to 140 mm of Hg in the foot pedal, so if a surge exist during the procedure the surgeon can increase the irrigation force by the simple touch of the footswitch to the right. With the AVGFI the surgeon has the capability to increase even more these values. A millipore filter is used again between the tubing and the air pump (Fig. 1.2).

STELLARIS PRESSURIZED INFUSION SYSTEM

Bausch and Lomb installed an air pump in their Stellaris machine in 2009. The advantage of this is that one has an internal gas forced infusion now as the air pump which was an external gas forced infusion system is now inside the machine (Fig. 1.3). Another advantage is there is a monitor in the panel of the machine and one can lower or raise the pressure of the air pump.

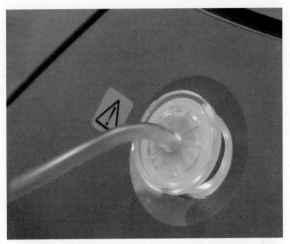

Figure 1.2 Millipore filter to connect the air pump to the tubing. Air pump in the Stellaris (Bausch and Lomb) machine

DISCUSSION

Surge is defined as the volume of the fluid forced out of the eye into the aspiration line at the instant of occlusion break. When the phacoemulsification handpiece tip is occluded, flow is interrupted and vacuum builds up to its preset values. Additionally the aspiration tubing may collapse in the presence of high vacuum levels. Emulsification of the occluding fragment clears the block and the fluid rushes into the aspiration line to neutralize the pressure difference created between the positive pressure in the anterior chamber and the negative pressure in the aspiration tubing. In addition, if the aspiration line tubing is not reinforced to prevent collapse (tubing compliance), the tubing, constricted during occlusion, then expands on occlusion break. These factors cause a rush of fluid from the anterior chamber into the phaco probe. The fluid in the anterior chamber is not replaced rapidly enough to prevent shallowing of the anterior chamber.

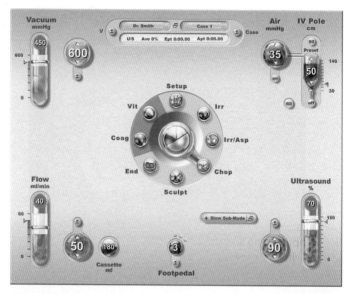

Figure 1.3 Stellaris (Bausch and Lomb) pressurized infusion system. Note in the upper right corner IV pole height in cm and next to it shows the air pump (gas forced infusion pressure) in mm of Hg

The maintenance of intraocular pressure (steady-state IOP)[2] during the entire procedure depends on the equilibrium between the fluid inflow and outflow. The steady state pressure level is the mean pressure equilibrium between inflow and outflow volumes. In most phacoemulsification machines, fluid inflow is provided by gravitational flow of the fluid from the balanced salt solution (BSS) bottle through the tubing to the anterior chamber. This is determined by the bottle height relative to the patient's eye, the diameter of the tubing and most importantly by the outflow of fluid from the eye through the aspiration tube and leakage from the wounds.[2]

The inflow volume can be increased by either increasing the bottle height or by enlarging the diameter of the inflow tube. The intraocular pressure increases by 10 mm Hg for every 15 centimeters increase in bottle height above the eye.[5]

High steady-state IOPs increase phaco safety by raising the mean IOP level up and away from zero, i.e. by delaying surge related anterior chamber collapse.[2]

Air pump increases the amount of fluid inflow thus making the steady-state IOP high. This deepens the anterior chamber, increasing the surgical space available for maneuvering and thus prevents complications like posterior capsular tears and corneal endothelial damage. The phenomenon of surge is neutralized by rapid inflow of fluid at the time of occlusion break. The recovery to steady-state IOP is so prompt that no surge occurs and this enables the surgeon to remain in foot position 3 through the occlusion break. High vacuum phacoemulsification/phakonit can be safely performed in hard brown cataracts using an air pump. Phacoemulsification or phakonit under topical or no anesthesia[6,7] can be safely done neutralizing the positive vitreous pressure occurring due to squeezing of the eyelids.

SUMMARY

The air pump is a new device, which helps to prevent surge. This prevents posterior capsular rupture, helps deepen the anterior chamber and makes phacoemulsification and phakonit a safe procedure even in hard cataracts.

REFERENCES

1. Kelman CD. Phacoemulsification and aspiration; a new technique of cataract removal; a preliminary report. Am J Ophthalmol. 1967; 64:23-5.
2. Wilbrandt RH. Comparative analysis of the fluidics of the AMO Prestige, Alcon Legacy, and Storz Premiere phacoemulsification systems. J Cataract Refract Surg. 1997;23:766-80.
3. Seibel SB. Phacodynamics. Thorofare, NJ, Slack Inc. 1995;54.
4. Fishkind WJ. The phaco machine : How and why it acts and reacts? In: Agarwal's Four Volume Textbook of Ophthalmology. Jaypee Brothers: New Delhi; 2000.

5. Seibel SB. The fluidics and physics of phaco. In: Agarwal, et al. (eds). Phacoemulsification, Laser Cataract Surgery and Foldable IOLs, 2nd edn. Jaypee Brothers: New Delhi. 2000.pp.45-54.

6. Agarwal, et al. No anesthesia cataract surgery with karate chop; In: Agarwal's Phacoemulsification, Laser Cataract Surgery and Foldable IOLs, 2nd edn. Jaypee Brothers: New Delhi. 2000.pp.217-26.

7. Agarwal, et al. Phakonit and laser phakonit.; In: Agarwal's Phacoemulsification, Laser Cataract Surgery and Foldable IOLs, 2nd edn. Jaypee Brothers: New Delhi. 2000.pp.204-16.

8. Agarwal A, Agarwal S, Agarwal A. Antichamber collapser. J Cataract and Refractive Surgery. 2002;28:1085.

9. Agarwal A, Agarwal S, Agarwal A. Phakonit: phacoemulsification through a 0.9 mm incision. J Cataract and Refractive Surgery. 2001; 27:1548-52.

10. Agarwal A, Trivedi RH, Jacob S, et al. Microphakonit: 700 micron cataract surgery. Clinical ophthalmology. 2007;1(3):323-5.

11. Agarwal A, Kumar DA, Jacob S, Agarwal A. In vivo analysis of wound architecture in 700 micron microphakonit surgery. J Cataract Refract Surg. 2008;34(9):1554-60.

2

Ophthalmic Viscosurgical Device

Priya Narang

INTRODUCTION

Ophthalmic viscosurgical devices (OVDs) are transparent, gel-like substances that have viscous and elastic properties. OVDs are used during surgery in order to maintain and preserve space, displace and stabilize tissue, and coat and protect tissue.

Ophthalmic viscosurgical devices are an essential part of cataract surgery (Figs 2.1 and 2.2). Apart from maintaining the anterior chamber depth and coating the corneal endothelium they are useful and applicable for various challenging scenarios encountered in the cataract surgery. There are different types of OVDs that are applicable in different scenarios to optimize the outcome of cataract surgery. They can be categorized according to their chemical constitution or according to their physical properties. OVDs have variety of uses in ophthalmic surgery that could be summarized in space creation, tissue stabilization and corneal endothelial cell protection.[1]

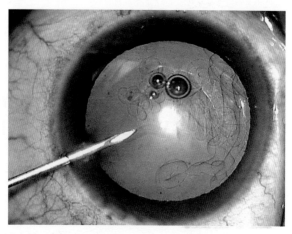

Figure 2.1 Viscoelastic injection: Viscoelastic is injected into the anterior chamber (AC). This makes the AC taut and thus helps in creating a well constructed main port

CHEMICAL CONSTITUTION

Hydroxy-Propyl Methyl Cellulose (HPMC)

It is a cellulose polymer modified by the addition of hydroxyl-propyl and methyl groups to increase the hydrophilic property of the material. Methylcellulose is a non-physiologic compound that is not metabolized intraocularly. It is eventually eliminated in the aqueous and is easily washed out of the eye.

Sodium Hyaluronate

Sodium hyaluronate is a biopolymer that occurs in many connective tissues throughout the body. It has a high molecular weight (2.5–4 million daltons) and low protein content and carries a single negative charge for the disaccharide unit. Hyaluronate has a half-life of approximately 1 day in aqueous and 3 days in vitreous.

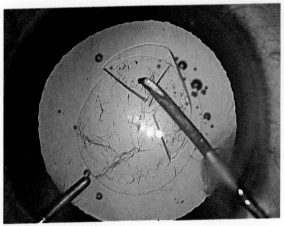

Figure 2.2 Rhexis: The tip of a 26 gauge is bent to form a cystitome. The bent tip is used to first create a nick on the anterior capsule horizontally outwards and then lift it up to create a flap. The tear follows the flap edge, hence the flap should be constantly adjusted to achieve the desired shape and size. Any vitreous thrust or positive intra-lenticular pressure can cause the rhexis margin to run towards the periphery. Hence, viscoelastic is reinjected as and when required to fill the AC and maintain a taut anterior capsule

Chondroitin Sulfate

Chondroitin sulfate is a viscoelastic biopolymer similar to hyaluronate but possessing a sulfated group with a double-negative charge. Chondroitin sulfate is commonly obtained from shark cartilage.

TYPES OF OVDs

Cohesive OVDs

They (Healon, Provisc, Amvisc, Amvisc plus) are long chain, high molecular weight, high viscosity substances that maintain space well at low shear rates, while at high shear rates they are easily displaced. The advantage is that they are easier to remove from the eye since they stick together and are aspirated as long pieces. Thus, there is less chance of retention and risk of an IOP spike. However, they have minimal coating ability and therefore afford less tissue protection during surgery. Thus, cohesives are used to expand the capsular bag for intraocular lens insertion at the end of cataract surgery.

Dispersive OVDs

They (viscoat, ocucoat) are short chain, low molecular weight, low viscosity substances with low surface tension. They have excellent coating properties and protection at high shear rates; however, they are more difficult to remove from the eye since they do not stick together and are aspirated in short fragments. Typically, dispersives remain in the eye during phacoemulsification to protect the endothelium from turbulent flow. Therefore, they have an increased risk of elevated IOP.

Viscoadaptive/ Viscodispersive OVDs

Viscoadaptive OVD[2] (Healon 5) is a long fragile chain, high molecular weight, super viscous substance that breaks at high shear rates. Therefore, it has properties of both cohesive and dispersive agents, mimicking cohesive OVDs at low flow and dispersive OVDs at high flow conditions. It is well retained in the eye and maintains space during high shear manipulations, but is also easily fractured so that it can coat well. It must be completely removed since it causes elevated IOP if left in the eye. DisCoVisc, a viscous dispersive agent, is another new OVD that is very good for stabilizing tissue, maintaining space at high shear rates, and coating the cornea. This biphasic nature has resulted in viscoadaptives being referred to as pseudodispersive in ophthalmic surgery because they are well retained in the anterior segment similar to dispersive OVDs.[3]

Since the cohesive and dispersive agents have different strengths and weaknesses, it is sometimes necessary to use both types of OVDs, either for different steps of a surgery or in combination for a single maneuver (i.e., soft shell technique for capsulorhexis or IOL insertion in which two different OVDs are layered one below the other to maximize the advantages of their different properties). Because the newer OVDs combine the advantages of the traditional agents, they may be more useful for a greater range of clinical applications.

Clinical Application

OVDs were first introduced to maintain space in the eye during the implantation of intraocular lenses. On the other hand, complications associated with the use of ophthalmic viscosurgical devices and their prevention have been discussed. Wound burns during phacoemulsification may occur and creating a fluid space around the phacoemulsification tip is necessary to avoid them. Its function during cataract surgery include maintaining the anterior chamber during the capsulorhexis and IOL insertion, preventing iris prolapse and trapping nuclear fragments, and protecting the corneal endothelium from turbulence, lens material, and ultrasound energy. They are also used to enlarge and stabilize the size of the pupil specifically in patients with small pupils or intraoperative floppy iris syndrome.

Key Points

- OVDs create a protective barrier.
- They help reduce free radicals.
- They create and maintain space within the anterior chamber and help in manipulation of tissues during surgery.
- They coat the surgical instruments and IOLs.
- Postoperative elevations of intraocular pressure have been reported and complete removal of the OVD at the end of surgery is the key factor to avoid these elevations.

REFERENCES

1. Arshinoff SA, Jafari M. New classification of ophthalmic viscosurgical devices–2005. J Cataract Refract Surg. 2005;31(11):2167-71.
2. Arshinoff SA. Why Healon5? The meaning of "viscoadaptive". Ophthalmic Pract. 1999;17:332-4.
3. Arshinoff SA, Wong E. Understanding, retaining, and removing dispersive and pseudodispersive ophthalmic viscosurgical devices. J Cataract Refract Surg. 2003;29(12):2318-23.

3

No-anesthesia Cataract Surgery with the Karate Chop Technique

Amar Agarwal

INTRODUCTION

On 13th June, 1998 at Ahmedabad, India the author at the Phaco and Refractive Surgery conference performed 'no anesthesia cataract surgery' for the first time in the world. This opened up various new concepts in cataract surgery[1-4] and the technique of karate chop was employed during the 'live surgery session'.

NUCLEUS REMOVAL TECHNIQUES

Since the introduction of phacoemulsification as an alternative to standard cataract extraction technique, surgeons throughout the world have been attempting to make this new procedure safer and easier to perform while assuring good visual outcome and patient recovery. The fundamental goal of phaco surgery is to remove the cataract with minimal disturbance to the eye using least number of surgical manipulations. Each maneuver should be performed with minimal force and maximal efficiency should be obtained.

The latest generation phaco procedures began with Dr. Howard Gimbel's "divide and conquer" nuclear fracture technique in which he simply split apart the nuclear rim. Since then we have evolved through the various techniques namely four quadrant cracking, chip and flip, spring surgery, stop and chop and phaco chop.

KARATE CHOP

Unlike the peripheral chopping of Nagahara or other stop and chop techniques we have developed a safer technique called "central anterior chopping" or "karate chop". In this method the phaco tip is embedded by a single burst of power in the central safe zone and after lifting the nucleus a little bit (to lessen the pressure on the posterior capsule) the chopper is used to chop the nucleus. In soft nuclei, it is very difficult to chop the nucleus. In most cases, one can take it out in toto. But if the patient is about 40 years of age then one might have to chop the nucleus. In such cases we embed the phaco probe in the nucleus and then with the left hand cut the nucleus as if we are cutting a piece of cake. This movement should be done three times in the same place. This will chop the nucleus.

SOFT CATARACTS

In soft cataracts, the technique is a bit different. We embed the phaco tip and then cut the nucleus as if we are cutting a piece of cake. This should be done 2–3 times in the same area so that the cataract gets cut. It is very tough to chop a soft cataract, so this technique helps in splitting the cataract.

AGARWAL CHOPPER

We have devised our own chopper. The other choppers, which cut from the periphery, are blunt choppers. Our chopper has a sharp cutting edge with a sharp point. The advantage of such a chopper is that the surgeon can chop in the center and need not go to the periphery.

In this method by going directly into the center of the nucleus, ultrasound energy can be imparted obviating the need of sculpting. The chopper always remains within the rhexis margin and never goes underneath the anterior capsule. Hence it is easy to work with even small pupils or glaucomatous eyes. Since we do not have to widen the pupil, there is less likelihood of tearing the sphincter and allowing prostaglandins to leak out and cause inflammation or cystoid macular edema. In this technique we can easily go into even hard nuclei on the first attempt.

KARATE CHOP TECHNIQUE

Incision

A temporal clear corneal section is made. If the astigmatism is plus at 90 degrees then the incision is made superiorly. First of all, a 26 G needle attached to a 1 mL syringe filled with viscoelastic is introduced inside the eye from the site where the side port incision is to be framed (Fig. 3.1). This distends the eye so that when a clear corneal incision is made, the eye remains inflated and a good corneal valve is fashioned. The eye is stabilized with a straight rod with the left hand while the right hand frames the clear corneal incision (Fig. 3.2).

When we started making the temporal incisions, we positioned ourselves temporally. The problem by this method is that, every time the microscope has to be turned which in turn would affect the cables connected to the video camera. Further the theater staff would get disturbed between right eye and left eye. To solve this problem, we then decided on a different strategy. We have operating trolleys on wheels. The patient is wheeled inside the operation theater and for the right eye the trolley is placed slightly obliquely so that the surgeon does not change his or her position. The surgeon stays at the 12 o'clock position. For the left eye the trolley with the patient is rotated horizontally so that the temporal portion of the left eye comes at 12 o'clock.

CAPSULORHEXIS

Capsulorhexis is then performed through the same incision (Fig. 3.3). While performing the rhexis it is important to note that the rhexis is

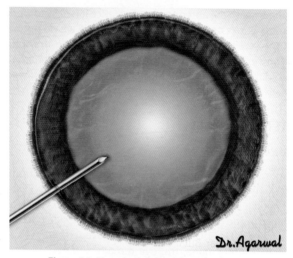

Figure 3.1 Viscoelastic being injected in the eye

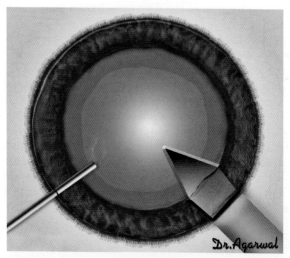

Figure 3.2 Clear corneal incision (*Note:* The straight road inside the eye in the left hand while the right hand fashions the clear corneal incision)

started from the center and the needle moved to the right and then downward. This is important because today concepts have changed of temporal and nasal. It is better to remember it as superior, inferior, right or left. If we would start the rhexis from the center and move it to the left then the weakest point of the rhexis is generally where you finish it. In other words, the point where you tend to lose the rhexis is near its completion. If you have done the rhexis from the center and moved to the left, then you might have an incomplete rhexis on the left-hand side either inferiorly or superiorly. Now, the phaco probe is always moved down and to the left. So every stroke of your hand can extend the rhexis posteriorly creating a posterior capsular rupture. Now, if we perform the rhexis from the center and move to the right and then push the flap inferiorly- then if we have an incomplete rhexis near the end of the rhexis it will be superiorly and to the right. Any incomplete rhexis can extend and create a posterior capsular tear. But in this case, the chances of survival are

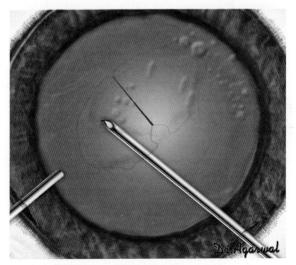

Figure 3.3 Capsulorhexis being done with a needle

better. This is because we are moving the phaco probe down and to the left, but the rhexis is incomplete up and to the right.

If you are a left handed person start the rhexis from the center and move to the left and then down.

HYDRODISSECTION

Hydrodissection is performed and the surgeon watches for the fluid wave to see that hydrodissection is complete. We do not perform hydro-delineation unless operating on a posterior polar cataract. In such a case only hydro-delineation is performed and not hydro-dissection. Viscoelastic is then introduced before inserting the phaco probe.

KARATE CHOP: TWO HALVES

Phaco probe is introduced through the incision slightly superior to the center of the nucleus (Fig. 3.4). At this point only ultrasound energy is applied till the phaco tip gets embedded in the nucleus . The direction of the phaco probe should be obliquely downwards toward the vitreous and not horizontally towards the iris. The settings at this stage are 70% phaco power, 24 mL/minute flow rate and 100 mm of Hg suction. By the time the phaco tip gets embedded in the nucleus the tip would have reached the middle of the nucleus. A zero degree or a 15 degree tip is preferred.

The surgeon switches to foot pedal position 2 so that only suction is being employed. The nucleus is lifted a little so that when pressure is applied on the nucleus with the chopper the direction of the pressure is downwards. In cases of hypermature cataracts where the posterior capsule is thin, lifting the nucleus decreases the pressure on posterior capsule and prevents an inadvertent rupture. With the help of the chopper, the nucleus is cut with a straight downward motion (Fig. 3.5) and the chopper is then moved to the left when the center of the nucleus is approached. In other words, the left hand moves the chopper like a laterally reversed 'L'.

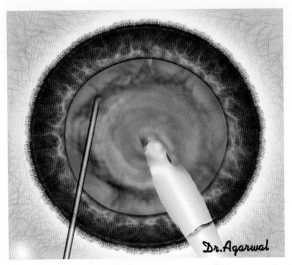

Figure 3.4 Phaco probe placed at the superior end of the capsulorhexis

Do Not Chop in the Periphery

Once the nucleus is cracked, split the nucleus till the center followed by 180 degrees rotation of the nucleus so that two halves of the nucleus are created. In brown cataracts, the nucleus is often difficult to crack and split. In such circumstances, the procedure has to be performed with lot of care and caution due to inherent weakness of the posterior capsule associated with dense cataract.

Karate Chop: Further Chopping

After achieving two halves of the nucleus, the surgeon places the phaco probe into one half of the nucleus (Fig. 3.6) with the direction of the probe being horizontal as shelfing has to be performed. Embed the probe and then slightly pull it a little bit so that the surgeon gets an extra bit of space for chopping. This helps prevent chopping the rhexis margin. Apply the force of the chopper downwards. Then move the chopper to the left so that the nucleus

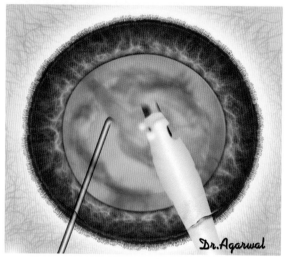

Figure 3.5 Phaco probe embedded in the nucleus. Start embedding from the superior end of the capsulorhexis. Left hand chops the nucleus and splits like a laterally reversed L, that is downwards and to the left

gets split. The surgeon should see the posterior capsule throughout the chopping procedure so that it is ensured that the nucleus is totally split. With the same method, create three quadrants in one half of the nucleus. Then make another three halves with the second half of the nucleus. Thus, the surgeon now has 6 quadrants or pie-shaped fragments. The settings at this stage are 50% phaco power, 24 mL/minute flow rate and 101 mm of Hg suction.

Remember 5 words: Embed, pull, chop, split and release.

Pulse Phaco

After all the pieces have been chopped, pull out each piece of the nucleus sequentially and in pulse phaco mode aspirate the pieces at the level of the iris. Do not work in the bag unless the cornea

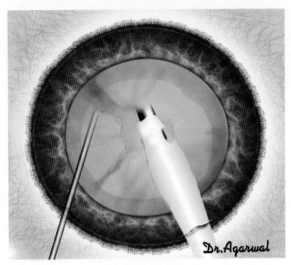

Figure 3.6 Phaco probe embedded in one half of the nucleus. Go horizontally and not vertically as the shelf of nucleus to has to be embedded. Chop and then split the nucleus

is preoperatively bad or the patient is very elderly. The air pump is advocated at this stage as surge is prevented and the chamber depth is maintained. The setting at this stage can be phaco power 50–30%, flow rate 24 mL and suction 100 mm of Hg.

Cortical Washing and Foldable IOL Implantation

The next step is to perform cortical washing (Fig. 3.7). Always try to remove the subincisional cortex first, as that is the most difficult. Note the left hand has the straight rod controlling the movements of the eye. If necessary use a bimanual irrigation aspiration technique. Then inject viscoelastic and implant the foldable IOL in the capsular bag.

Stromal Hydration

At the end of the procedure, inject the BSS inside the lips of the clear corneal incision. This will create a stromal hydration at the wound. The incision site looks apparently chalky white, which usually disappear within next 4–5 hours. Stromal hydration helps to seal the wound site in a better way.

No Pad, Subconjunctival Injections

No subconjunctival injections or eye pad is applied. The patient is seen the next day and after a month glasses are prescribed.

NO ANESTHESIA CATARACT SURGERY

The importance and validity of topical anesthesia in cataract surgery always created an enigmatic penumbra in our minds. So we then

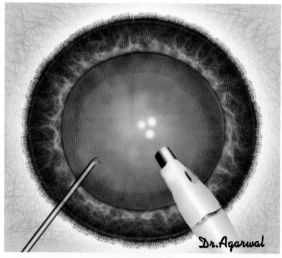

Figure 3.7 Cortical aspiration completed. Note the straight rod in the left hand which helps control the movements of the eye

decided to operate patients without any topical xylocaine drops. To our surprise, the patients never complained of pain which is quite paradoxical to the fact that anesthesia is always needed to perform a surgery. The point of caution to be mentioned is that at no point during the surgery, a surgeon should touch the conjunctiva with a forceps or any other instrument. At our center, after inflating the eye with viscoelastic from a side port incision, we use a straight rod that is passed inside the eye to stabilize it when capsulorhexis is being performed. Francisco Gutierrez-Carmona from Spain modified the technique using cold fluid and has termed it as cryoanalgesia.

AIR PUMP TO PREVENT SURGE

One of the main bugbears of phacoemulsification is Surge.[1] As the nuclear piece gets occluded in the phaco tip during emulsification, surge is often induced. Various methods have been employed to overcome this issue and some Phaco machines have been devised to solve this problem too. Many surgeons use an anterior chamber maintainer to infuse more fluid into the eye. With the employment of an anterior chamber maintainer, a separate side port incision has to be framed. In other words, three ports are fashioned which become quite cumbersome during the "no-anesthesia cataract surgery". Another method to solve surge is to use more of phacoaspiration and chop the nuclear pieces with the left hand (non-dominant hand). The problem is that in a case of hard brown cataract, phacoaspiration does not suffice well.

Surge occurs when an occluded fragment is held by high vacuum and is then abruptly aspirated with a burst of ultrasound. Sequentially, the fluid from the anterior chamber rushes into the phaco tip and this leads to a collapse of the anterior chamber. Sunita Agarwal thought of a method to solve surge using an air pump.

CONCLUSION

As in any other field, progress is inevitable in ophthalmology more so in refractive surgery. We have started to look on cataract surgery as a craft and should constantly try to improvise our craftsmanship and strive towards excellence every day. By doing so, we will be able to provide good vision to more people than any one dared dream a few decades ago.

Key Points

- In "Central anterior chopping" or "karate chop" the phaco tip is embedded by a single burst of power in the central safe zone and after lifting the nucleus a little bit (to lessen the pressure on the posterior capsule) the chopper is used to chop the nucleus.
- In soft cataracts, the technique is a bit different. Embed the phaco tip and then cut the nucleus as if cutting a piece of cake. This should be done 2–3 times in the same area so that the cataract gets cut.
- The Agarwal chopper is a sharp chopper. It has a sharp cutting edge. It also has a sharp point. The advantage of such a chopper is that you can chop in the center and need not go to the periphery.
- Never use any one-tooth forceps to stabilize the eye. Instead use a straight rod, which is passed inside the eye to stabilize it when performing capsulorhexis, etc.
- Routinely use the air pump to solve the problem of surge.

REFERENCES

1. Agarwal S, Agarwal A, Sachdev MS, Mehta KR, Fine HI, Agarwal A. Phacoemulsification, Laser Cataract Surgery & Foldable IOL's; 2nd edn. Jaypee Brothers Medical Publishers; 2000, Delhi, India.
2. Agarwal A, Agarwal S, Agarwal A. No anesthesia cataract surgery with the karate chop technique; In Amar Agarwal's Presbyopia: A surgical textbook; Slack Incorporated. 2002; USA; pages 177-85.
3. Agarwal A, Agarwal S, Agarwal A. No anesthesia cataract and clear lens extraction with karate chop; In: Agarwal's Phaco, Phakonit and laser Phaco: A quest for the best; Highlights of Ophthalmology. 2002; Panama; pages 113-20.
4. Agarwal A, Agarwal S, Agarwal A. No anesthesia cataract and clear lens extraction with karate chop ; In Boyd-Agarwal's Lasik and beyond Lasik; Highlights of Ophthalmology. 2001; Panama; pages 451-62.

4

Phaco in Subluxated Cataracts

Amar Agarwal, Priya Narang

INTRODUCTION

The surgical management of cataract associated with zonular dialysis is a real challenge for the ophthalmic surgeon. Due to recent advances in equipment and instrumentation, better surgical techniques and understanding of the fluidics, the surgeon is able to perform relatively safe cataract surgery in presence of compromised zonules. Implantation of a capsular tension ring can stabilize a loose lens and allow the surgeon to complete phacoemulsification and IOL implantation.

HISTORY

Insertion of a ring into the capsular bag fornix (equator) to support the zonular apparatus was first described by Hara and coauthors in 1991.[1] Hara et al. introduced the concept of "equator ring", "endocapsular ring" or "capsular tension ring (CTR)". In 1993, the first capsular tension ring (CTR) for use in humans was designed.[2] In 1994, Nagamato and Bissen-Miyajima[3] suggested using an open polymethyl methacrylate (PMMA) ring to provide adaptability.

ADVANTAGES

This technique offers four main advantages:

1. The capsular zonular anatomical barrier is partially reformed, so that vitreous herniation to the anterior chamber during surgery is reduced or even avoided.
2. A taut capsular equator offers counter traction for all traction maneuvers, making them easier to perform and decreasing the risk of extending the zonular dialysis. The great advantage of using the capsular ring during the phacoemulsification rather than after, just to center the lens is a great deal safer. Any force that is transmitted to the capsule is not applied directly to the adjacent zonules, but rather distributed circumferentially to the entire zonular apparatus.
3. The necessary capsular support for an in the bag, centered implant is obtained.
4. The capsular bag maintains its shape and does not collapse, which can lead to proliferation and migration of epithelial cells, development of capsular fibrosis syndrome and late IOP decentration.

DESIGNS AND DESCRIPTIONS

The capsular tension ring is made of one piece polymethyl methacrylate (PMMA) and is available in different sizes depending on their use in patients with emmetropia, low or high myopia. An injector is also present for loading the ring. The original capsular tension ring, with characteristic eyelets on both ends is marketed by Morcher company in co-operation with Dr Mitchel Morcher. Meanwhile, various similar products are being marketed (e.g. by ophtec physiol, corneal, IOL tech, Acrimed, Rayner, Hanita, Lens Tec.) As a standard capsular tension ring, 12.0/10.0 mm diameter ring (Morcher type 14) and the 13.0/11.0 mm diameter ring (ophtec 13/11) are the most commonly used by surgeons. Morcher type 14 are for normal axial length eyes, while type 14A and 14C are for myopic eyes.

The modifications used, by Morcher, include two types of capsular tension rings with iris shields (Type L and G, with integrated iris shields of 60 and 90 degrees, respectively) and two types of capsular bending rings (CBRs) designed to prevent capsule opacification (type E and F).These modified versions incorporate fixation elements that allow the surgeon to suture the ring to the scleral wall, through the ciliary sulcus, without violating the capsular ring.[4]

Special Designs for Suturing in Severe Zonular Dehiscence

In cases where severe or progressive zonular dehiscence is present implantation of the capsular tension ring alone may not be adequate. This may lead to severe postoperative capsular bag shrinkage as well as IOL decentration and pseudophakodonesis.[5] Also complete luxation of the bag along with the capsular tension ring and the IOL cannot be excluded.

A modified design developed by Cionni with a fixation hook for severe or progressive cases of zonular deficiency[6] solves this problem. The hook is kept opposite to the meridian of decentration and is pulled peripherally using a transscleral fixation suture, to counteract capsular bag decentration and tilt. In severe cases two such rings or the two hooked model can be used. However the Cionni ring has its limitations like difficulty to implant if the capsulorhexis is small and in such cases the hook may even drag on the edge of the anterior capsule, and as the fixation plane is anterior to the anterior capsule, it may lead to iris chafing leading to pigment dispersion and chronic uveitis.

An alternative is to fix the ring by guiding the needle of the scleral suture through the equator of the capsular bag, just inside the capsular tension ring.[7] This technique has to be completed as a one step procedure because the suture may cheese-wire through both capsules leaving along the equator.

Another alternative in cases of severe decentration is to make a small equatorial capsulorhexis through which a standard capsular tension ring can be inserted. A scleral suture can then be passed around the exposed capsular tension ring which is then used to center the lens before capsulorhexis.

INDICATIONS

The indication for use of capsular tension ring is in all cases of subluxation of lens (Table 4.1) ranging from the common ones like traumatic displacement (mechanical or surgical), Marfan's syndrome, pseudoexfoliation syndrome and hypermature cataract to the rare ones like aniridia and intraocular tumors.

APPLICATIONS

Zonular Dehiscence

The efficacy of the capsular tension ring in managing zonular dialysis has been demonstrated in vitro[8,9] depending on where the zonular defect presents. The capsular tension ring may be inserted at any stage of cataract procedure. By reestablishing the capsules contour, the capsular tension ring protects the capsular fornix from being aspirated, avoiding consecutive zonular dialysis extension, irrigation fluid running behind the capsular diaphragm with the posterior capsule bulging, and vitreous prolapse into the anterior chamber with possible aspiration. With pre-existing zonular defects such as those caused by blunt trauma, the capsular tension ring is inserted before phacoemulsification is started.

Zonular Weakness

Ocular and systemic conditions may result in a zonular weakness that may be profound and progressive. Pseudoexfoliation syndrome with or without glaucoma and Marfan's syndrome are the most common causes. If zonular weakness is profound the capsular tension ring is implanted before the cataract is emulsified and a 10-0 nylon anchoring suture may be temporarily threaded through the eyelets so as to remove the capsular tension ring if the zonules fail during surgery.

TABLE 4.1 Etiology of subluxated lenses

- Isolated ocular abnormality
  - Simple ectopia lentis
  - Simple microspherophakia
  - Spontaneous, late subluxation of lens
- Associated with other ocular abnormality
  - Aniridia
  - Ectopia lentis et pupillae
  - Uveal coloboma
  - Cornea plana
- Associated with heritable systemic syndromes
  - Marfan's syndrome
  - Homocystinuria
  - Weill-Marchesani syndrome
  - Ehler-Danlos syndrome
  - Rieger's syndrome
  - Hyperlysinemia
  - Sulfite oxidase deficiency
  - Sturge-Weber syndrome
  - Pflander's syndrome
  - Crouzon's syndrome
  - Sprengel's anomaly
  - Oxycephaly
- Associated with other ocular conditions
  - Mature or hypermature cataract
  - Mechanical stretching of zonules
    - Buphthalmos
    - Staphylomas
    - Ectasias of globe
    - High myopia
    - Perforation of large central corneal ulcer
  - Pull on zonules
    - Cyclitic inflammatory adhesions
    - Eales disease
    - Persistent hyperplastic primary vitreous
    - Intraocular tumors
    - Retinal detachment
  - Degeneration of zonules
    - Uveitis
    - Retinitis pigmentosa
    - Chalcosis
    - Prolonged silicone oil tamponade
    - High myopia
    - Hypermature cataract
- Traumatic subluxation/dislocation and surgical trauma

In pseudoexfoliation syndrome, the anterior capsule may contract excessively after in the bag IOL placement (capsular phimosis). This can be prevented by providing a locking mechanism that would prevent the eyelets from overlapping, suturing together the two eyelets together or by using two larger implants. This can be supplemented by meticulously polishing the anterior capsule leaf overlapping the implant.

In case of Marfan's syndrome the zonules may be disintegrated or elongated while the remaining may be still functional, giving rise to lens decentration, which may be progressive. In case of Weill-Marchesani syndrome, microspherophakia and zonular degeneration may occur. Secondary scleral suturing to remedy IOL decentration and tilt may be useful in such cases.[7]

Use of prolonged silicone oil tamponade may lead to progressive zonular atrophy and emulsified oil or oil bubble gaining access into the anterior chamber spontaneously or during the cataract surgery. In such cases a large capsular tension ring should be implanted before phacoemulsification is done.

LENS COLOBOMA

A colobomatous lens (Fig. 4.1) is due to defective or absent segment of zonules resulting in a notch in the lens. It is a misnomer in that there is no actual lenticular substance missing. There is just a retraction of a crystalline area due to localized loss of tension on the lens capsule. Intact zonules are often seen in this area and therefore a localized area of defective ciliary body or zonules may lead to localized loss of traction on the lens capsule. It may occur along with a ciliary body coloboma. Lens coloboma is, therefore, more accurately referred to as *coloboma of the zonule and/or ciliary body*.

Surgery in Lens Coloboma

Surgery is done using a capsular tension ring (CTR) which forms the capsular fornix (Figs 4.2 to 4.4). The CTR which was first started by T Hara protects against capsular fornix aspiration, consecutive

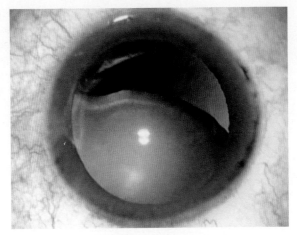

Figure 4.1 Lens coloboma

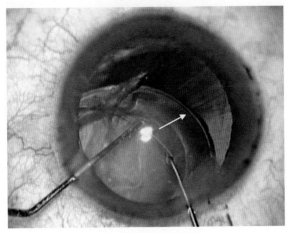

Figure 4.2 Endocapsular ring implantation

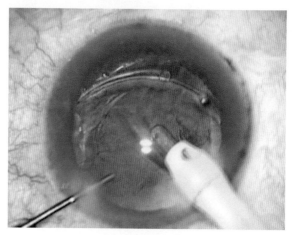

Figure 4.3 Cortical aspiration

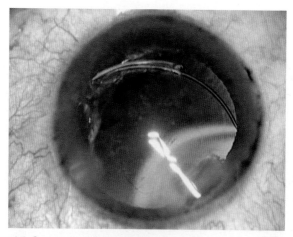

Figure 4.4 Cortex removed. (*Note:* The lens coloboma and endocapsular ring. At this stage one can implant the foldable IOL comfortably)

zonular dialysis, irrigation fluid flowing behind the capsule, vitreous herniating into the anterior chamber, IOL decentration, and capsular phimosis. Minimal mydriasis or reactive miosis may be a problem. Conventional approaches to deal with normally positioned small pupils and cataract surgery may be used, such as mechanical stretching, iris retractors, or multiple sphincterotomies. Vitreous loss may occur secondary to prolapse through the coloboma in the presence of an intact capsule. Giant retinal tears also occur with isolated lens coloboma. A large optic IOL is advisable for better visualization of the posterior segment, which is at greater risk of potential retinal detachment and also for optimal centration of the optic relative to the ectopic pupil. Aberration free or aspheric IOLs may also be preferable in these eyes to decrease the effect of lens decentration on vision. A silicone IOL is not advised in case a complex retinal detachment occurs that requires the use of silicone oil.

Technique

Anesthesia

Both general and peribulbar anesthesia are suitable for creation of scleral windows and transscleral suturing of the capsular ring or of the IOL if necessary. Special mention is required about 1% intracameral lidocaine. There is a risk of its passage through the zones lacking zonular fibers, and transitory loss of sight resulting from retinal toxicity, as described in cases of capsular ruptures.[10]

Incisions

The first step is to make an incision in the eye which has a subluxated cataract. A needle with viscoelastic is injected inside the eye in the area where the second site is made. This will distend the eye so that when you make a clear corneal incision, the eye will be tense and one can create a good valve. Now use a straight rod to stabilize the eye with the left hand. With the right hand make the clear corneal incision.

Capsulorhexis

Commencing capsulorhexis is difficult because of capsular instability. It is better to begin the capsulorhexis in the area where the zonules is whole and where the capsule offers sufficient resistance. If vitreous is present in the anterior chamber, the gel must be first isolated and vitrectomy should be performed if required. After the vitreous has been removed from the anterior chamber, a viscoelastic preferably dispersive is inserted by first covering the zone. Capsulorhexis can be performed after the zone of zonular dehiscence and iridocrystalline diaphragm have been stabilized. Do not use trypan blue in such cases as the trypan blue will go into the vitreous cavity through the zonular dehiscence and make the whole vitreous cavity blue. This will make visualization difficult in surgery. Completion of rhexis can be done using an intraocular rhexis forceps.

Hydrodissection and Hydrodelineation

Hydromaneuvers should be performed meticulously to ensure correct freeing of the lens nucleus. The hydrodissection cannula should be inserted in the direction of the zone of disinsertion rather than in the opposite direction, which would enlarge the disinsertion. Viscoelastic may be required to separate the nucleus and cortical material and also to separate the cortex from the lens capsule.

Implantation of Capsular Ring

Mostly capsular tension rings can be easily inserted in the capsular bag if it is well expanded with viscoelastic. The instruments used to implant a capsular tension ring include Kelman-McPherson type forceps special injectors (marketed by Ophtec and Geuder suitable for both Ophtec and Morcher CTRs and the one developed by Menapace and Nishi for use with CBR, Geuder Co.) and last but not the least a guiding suture.

Phacoemulsification

Nuclear phacoemulsificaton can be performed using coaxial phaco or bimanual phaco/phakonit in the bag or out of the bag, depending on the surgeon's preference. In general, phacoemulsification in these situations may be considered a safe proposition if performed in a proper way.

Cortical Aspiration

When performing automated aspiration, movements of the tip should not be radial because of the risk of traction on the ring and the capsular bag.

Implantation of the Intraocular Lens

It is desirable to implant a larger diameter lens to minimize symptoms if lens decentration were to occur. The foldable lens is loaded and implanted in the capsular bag followed by viscoelastic removal. In either case, rotational maneuvers must be avoided or minimized.[11]

CIONNI'S RING

If the lens continues to remain decentered after CTR insertion, a flexible nylon iris hook is used to engage the rhexis margin through a paracentesis opposite to the direction of subluxation. This gives capsular support till the end of surgery at which time a transscleral fixation of one haptic of the IOL can be done for its centration.

When zonular dehiscence is large in extent or progressive in nature, capsular bag shrinkage resulting in IOL decentration and pseudophakodonesis may occur even after a successful surgery with capsular ring. Complete luxation of the bag and its contents has also been reported. For such cases, Cionni's modified design with a fixation hook is a good solution (Fig. 4.5). The hook is kept in the area of dialysis and is pulled peripherally using a transscleral fixation suture, to counteract capsular bag decentration and tilt.

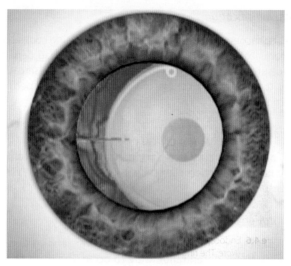

Figure 4.5 Cionni's ring

In severe cases, two such rings or the two hooked model can be used. If normal endocapsular ring is used the ring and the IOL might not be in the correct position (Fig. 4.6). An alternative in cases of severe decentration (Fig. 4.7) is to make a small equatorial capsulorhexis through which a standard capsular tension ring can be inserted. A scleral suture can then be passed around the exposed capsular tension ring which is then used to center the lens before capsulorhexis. Peribulbar anesthesia is suitable for creation of scleral windows and transscleral suturing of the capsular ring or of the IOL if necessary.

IKE SEGMENTS

Ike Ahmed designed the Ike segments which can be used for small segments.

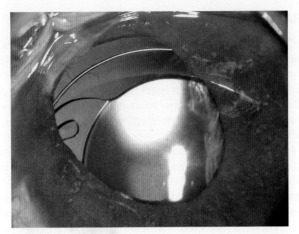

Figure 4.6 Endocapsular ring implanted without suturing to the sclera
(*Note:* The ring and IOL are not in proper place)

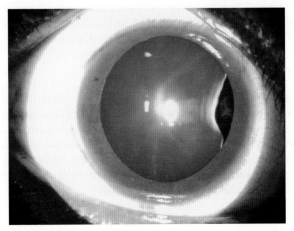

Figure 4.7 Lens coloboma

ASSIA'S CAPSULE ANCHOR

The Capsular Anchor (Hanita lenses, Kibbutz Hanita, Israel) is a novel device for the management of subluxation of the lens associated with moderate to severe zonular dehiscence or weakness. This was designed by Ehud Assia from Israel. It is a polymethyl methacrylate (PMMA) intraocular, uni-planer implant, inserted into the capsular bag after capsulorhexis is performed. An intact anterior continuous curvilinear capsulorhexis (ACCC) is a pre-requisite for a safe use of the Anchor. The two lateral arms of the device are inserted behind the anterior lens capsule whereas the central rod is placed in front of the capsule (Fig. 4.8). A 10-0, or preferably 9-0, prolene suture is used to fixate the Anchor to the scleral wall. The suture is either threaded through the hole in the base of the device or wraps around the neck of the anterior rod. A temporary safety suture can be used to prevent falling of the device during surgical procedures through the large zonular defect, especially if anterior vitrectomy was also performed. The Anchor is usually inserted prior to removal of the lens material. Repositioning and stabilization of the lens capsule significantly facilitate phacoemulsification or aspiration of the lens material and implantation of a PC-IOL (Figs 4.9A and B).

CONCEPT

The concept of the Capsular Anchor is different than that of the modified capsular rings. The later stabilize the capsular equator (the entire circumference—MCTR, or partial circumference—CTS). The Anchor clips a segment of the anterior capsule, and supports only a limited portion of the lens equator. A conventional capsular tension ring can be used in conjunction with the Anchor to reform the round contour of the capsular equator.

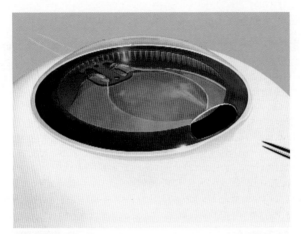

Figure 4.8 Schematic illustration of the capsular Anchor. The 2 lateral arms are located behind the anterior capsule. The anterior central rod is placed in front of the capsule

Keypoints with the use of Capsular Tension Rings

- Use a high viscosity viscoelastic.
- Make the incision at a meridian with no zonular dialysis, in order to avoid damage to zonular fibers with the movement of the phaco tip.
- Perform slow-motion phaco, with low flow rate, low vacuum, and low infusion bottle height.
- Emulsification can be done in the bag when the nucleus is soft and in the anterior chamber if the nucleus is hard thereby avoiding as much stress as possible to the already damaged zonular apparatus.
- Perform a careful two port anterior vitrectomy with lax infusion bottle and low aspiration pressure when necessary.
- Try to place IOL haptics in the meridian of the zonular disinsertion.
- IOL stability must be checked at the end of the surgery, both in the frontal and saggital plane in order to consider if suturing one haptic to the sulcus is necessary.[6]

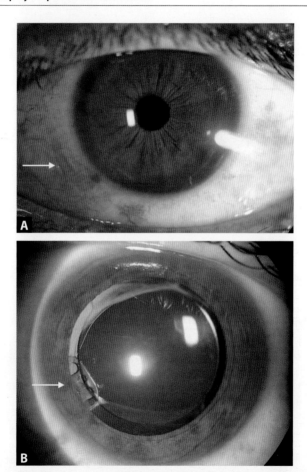

Figures 4.9A and B Subluxated case, 3 months postoperatively: A. Nondilated pupil is round, suture is buried under the conjuctiva (arrow); B. Dilated pupil—the Anchor fixates the inferonasal anterior capsule to the scleral wall (arrow), PC-IOL is well centered

Special Conditions

- *Coloboma shield for large sector iris defects or iridodialysis:* Tinted capsular tension ring with an integrated 60 to 90 degree sector shield designed by Rasch can be used to protect against glare and/or monocular diplopia (Morcher L and G).The capsular tension ring can be placed to cover sector iris defects and /or coloboma. If more than 90 degrees of defect is present then more than one capsular tension ring can be used.[4]
- *Multisegmented coloboma ring for aniridia:* This multisegmented ring designed by Rasch (Morcher type 50 C) is used in combination with the one of the same kind so that the interspaces of the first ring are covered by the sector shields of the second forming a contiguous artificial iris (Fig. 4.10).

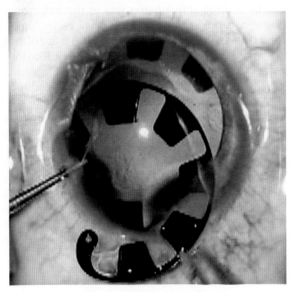

Figure 4.10 Aniridia rings being implanted

- *Anterior eye wall resection for uveal melanoma or other intraocular malignancy:* A combined use of a standard and coloboma capsular tension ring is advocated in cataract surgery after anterior eye wall resection for intraocular malignancy like uveal melanoma. Uveal tumors involving the anterior segment of the eye may need uveal resection resulting in large iris coloboma and zonular dehiscence. The crystalline lens may be cataractous or may become opaque after the surgery of the tumor requiring its removal sooner or later. For technical approach intracapsular cataract extraction was considered previously, but the combined use of a standard and coloboma capsular tension ring may help preserve the capsular bag and cover the iris defects.

- *Along with primary posterior capsulorhexis:* For pre-existing central capsule fibrosis or as a general preventive measure against capsule opacification.[12] As the capsular tension ring is in place, vector forces during primary posterior capsulorhexis can be controlled in a better way as the ring stretches the posterior capsule, giving uniform radial vector forces. As the capsular tension ring is in place distortion in shape of the primary posterior capsulorhexis can be avoided and folds on the capsule caused by traction due to oversized and rigid lens loop can be prevented, which allows closer and perfect apposition of the posterior capsule with the optic of the IOL thereby preventing lens epithelial cells (LECs) from entering the retrolental space in the posterior capsulorhexis margin and thus preventing the secondary primary posterior capsulorhexis closure.

- *In combined cataract and vitreous surgery:* When the capsular tension ring is in place, the posterior capsule remains uniformly distended and a perfect peripheral view is possible. Also as the capsular tension ring is in place silicone oil can be removed through the same phaco incision from the primary posterior capsulorhexis, which can be performed in a controlled manner with the capsular tension ring in place.

- *As a tool to measure capsular bag circumference:* The capsular tension ring in vivo can be visualized gonioscopically from a well dilated pupil. The distance between the eyelets can be determined by adjusting the width of the slitbeam of the slitlamp to fill in the space between the eyelets which can be read out on the slitlamp directly. This capsular bag biometry can be used for quantifying in vivo capsular bag circumference[13] and capsular bag shrinkage dynamics.[14]

- *For prevention of posterior capsular opacification:* Theoretically the lesser the space in between the lens optic and the posterior capsule the lesser are the chances of lens epithelial cells from migrating behind the optic, i.e. no space no cells. When the capsular bending ring is in place, this interspace is less common and if present less in amount as compared to without a capsular bending ring. Also by keeping the anterior capsule away from the posterior capsule, myofibroblastic transdifferentiation of lens epithelial cells on the anterior capsule edge and back surface can be prevented. The capsular bending ring is an open, band shaped polymethyl methacrylate ring measuring 11 mm in diameter with pretension (13 mm diameter when open), 0.2 mm in thickness, and 0.7 mm in thickness.

  The ring is minimally polished to keep the edges sharp and rectangular, facilitating the creation of a sharp, discontinuous band in the equatorial capsule. A crooked islet is located at both the ring ends to prevent spearing of the capsular fornix and to facilitate manipulation during insertion. The capsular bending ring reduces anterior capsular fibrosis and shrinkage as well as posterior capsular opacification. The ring may be useful in patients who are at high risk of developing eye complications from opacification that require Nd:YAG laser capsulotomy, in those expected to have vitreoretinal surgery and photocoagulation, and in cases of pediatric cataract.[15]

GLUED IOL

The latest technique for managing subluxated cataracts or colobomas is the use of the glued IOL (Chapter 14). In this a lensectomy vitrectomy is done and the lens removed totally. Then a glued IOL is implanted. The advantage is that pseudoexfoliations are progressive conditions and with glued IOL there is no problem (Figs 4.11A and B).

SUMMARY

Capsular tension rings or endocapsular rings have solved the problems of phaco in subluxated cataracts. They have made life much easier for the cataract surgeon.

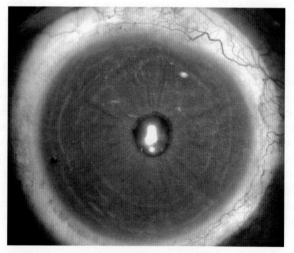

Figure 4.11A Glued IOL: A. Glued IOL done in right eye one and half year postoperative

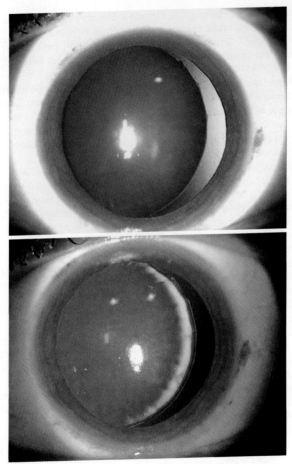

Figure 4.11B Subluxated cataract in left eye

REFERENCES

1. Hara T, Hara T, Yamada Y. "Equatorial ring" for maintainance of the completely circular contour of the capsular bag equator after cataract removal. Ophthalmic Surg. 1991;22:358-9.

2. Hara T, Hara T, Sakanishi K, Yamada Y. Efficacy of equator rings in a experimental rabbit study. Arch Ophthalmol. 1995;113:1060-5.

3. Nagamoto T, Bissen-Miyajima H. A ring to support the capsular bag after continuous curvilinear capsulorhexis Cataract Refract Surg. 1994;20:417-20.

4. Rupert Menapace, Oliver Findl, Michael Georgopoulos, Georg Rainer, Clemens Vass, Karin Schmetter. The capsular tension ring: Designs, applications, and techniques. J Cataract Refract Surg. 2000;898-912.

5. Nishi O, Hishi K, Sakanishi K, Yamada Y. Explantation of endocapsular posterior chamber lens after spontaneous posterior dislocation. J Cataract Refract Surg. 1996;22:272-5.

6. Groessl SA, Anderson CJ. Capsular tension ring in a patient with Weill-Marchesani syndrome. J Cataract and Refract Surg. 1998;24:1164-5.

7. Fischel JD, Wishart MS. Spontaneous complete dislocation of the lens in pseudoexfoliation syndrome. Eur J Implant Refract Surg. 1995;7:31-3.

8. Sun R, Gimbel HV. In vitro evaluation of the efficacy of the capsular tension ring for managing zonular dialysis in cataract surgery. Ophthalmic Surg Lasers. 1998;29:502-5.

9. Gimble HV, Sun R, Heston JP. Management of zonular dialysis in phacoemulsification and IOL implantation using the capsular tension ring. Ophthalmic Surg Lasers. 1997;28:273-81.

10. Gills J, Fenzil R. Intraocular lidocaine causes transient loss of vision in small number of cases. Ocular Surgery News. 1996.

11. Sunita Agarwal, Athiya Agarwal, Mahipal S Sachdev, Keiki R Mehta, I Howard Fine, Amar Agarwal: Phacoemulsification, Laser Cataract Surgery and Foldable IOL's; 2nd edn. Jaypee Brothers Medical Publishers, Delhi, India. 2000.

12. Van Cauwenberge F, Rakic J-M,Galand A. Complicated poserior capsulorhexis: etiology, management, and outcome. Br J Ophthalmol. 1997;81:195-8.

13. Vass C, Menapace R, Schametter K, et al. Prediction of pseudophacic capsular bag diameter on biometric variables. J Cataract Refract Surg. 1999;25:1376-81.

14. Strenn K, Menapace R,Vass C. Capsular bag shrinkage after implantation of an open loop silicone lens and a polymethyl methacrylate capsule tension ring. J Cataract Refract Surg. 1997;23:1543-7.

15. Okihiro Nishi, Kayo Nishi, Rupert Menaopace, Junsuke Akura. Capsular bending ring to prevent posterior capsule opacification: 2 year follow up. J Cataract Refract Surg. 2001;27:1359-65.

5

Mature Cataracts

Priya Narang, Amar Agarwal

INTRODUCTION

One of the biggest bugbears for a phaco surgeon is to perform a rhexis in a mature cataract (Figs 5.1 and 5.2). Once one performs rhexis in mature and hypermature cataracts, then phaco can be done in these cases and a foldable IOL implanted.

RHEXIS IN MATURE CATARACTS

Various techniques are present which can help one perform rhexis in mature cataracts.

- One should use a good operating microscope. If the operating microscope is good one can faintly see the outline of the rhexis.
- Use of an endoilluminator. While one is performing the rhexis with the right hand (dominant hand), in the left hand (non-dominant hand) one can hold an endoilluminator. By adjusting the endoilluminator in various positions, one can complete the rhexis as the edge of the rhexis can be seen.

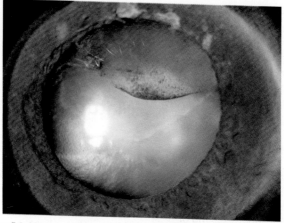

Figure 5.1 Mature cataract. It is difficult to visualize the rhexis in such cases. So we need to stain the anterior capsule with a dye

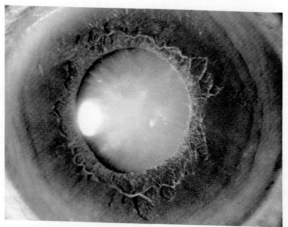

Figure 5.2 Mature cataract (*Note:* Vitreous is there anterior to the cataract)

- Use of a forceps. A forceps is easier to use than a needle especially in mature cataracts. One can use a good rhexis forceps to complete the rhexis.
- Use of paraxial light.

But with all these techniques, still one is not very sure of completing a rhexis in all cases. Many times if the rhexis is incomplete, one might have to convert to an extracapsular cataract extraction to prevent a posterior capsular rupture or nucleus drop.

Trypan Blue

The solution to this problem is to have a dye, which stains the anterior capsule. This dye is Trypan blue (Fig. 5.3). Each mL contains 0.6 mg Trypan blue, 1.9 mg of sodium mono-hydrogen orthophosphate, 0.3 mg of sodium di-hydrogen orthophosphate, 8.2 mg of sodium chloride, sodium hydroxide for adjusting the pH and water for injection. There are many other companies making this dye.

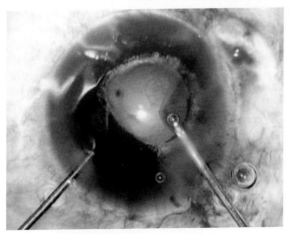

Figure 5.3 Trypan blue stained anterior capsule

ICG

Indocyanine green (ICG) is available in the U.S. It comes as a lyophilized compound, which must first be dissolved in 0.5 cc of sterile diluent supplied by the manufacturer. It is then further diluted with 4.5 cc of BSS plus (Alcon) immediately prior to use. This creates a 270 mOsm, 0.5% concentration. ICG creates a pale green staining of the capsule, which is gone by the conclusion of the case. One slight disadvantage is that the dye is lyophilized and larger particles often remain suspended in the mixture.

TECHNIQUE

We always tend to perform a temporal clear corneal incision. If the astigmatism is plus at 90 degrees then the incision is made superiorly. Trypan blue can be injected under air or directly into the anterior chamber. Trypan blue is withdrawn from the vial into a syringe. This is then injected by a cannula into the anterior chamber between the air bubble and the lens capsule. It is kept like that for a minute or two for staining of the anterior capsule to occur. Next viscoelastic is injected into the anterior chamber to remove the air bubble and the Trypan blue.

Now, rhexis is started with a needle. One can use a forceps also. We prefer to use a needle as it gives better control on the size of the rhexis. Note the left hand holding a rod stabilizing the eye while the rhexis is being performed. The rhexis is continued with the needle. Note the contrast between the capsule, which has been stained, and the cortex, which is not stained. The rhexis is continued and finally completed.

Hydrodissection is then done. One will not be able to see the fluid wave in such cases as the cataract is very dense. In such cases a simple way is to see if the lens comes up anteriorly a little bit. This will indicate hydrodissection being completed. One can also test this by rotating the nucleus before starting phaco.

We then insert the Phaco probe through the incision slightly superior to the center of the nucleus. At that point apply ultrasound and see that the phaco tip gets embedded in the nucleus. The direction of the phaco probe should be obliquely downwards toward the vitreous and not horizontally towards the iris. Then only the nucleus will get embedded. The settings at this stage are 80% phaco power, 24 mL/minute flow rate and 101 mm of Hg suction. By the time the phaco tip gets embedded in the nucleus the tip would have reached the middle of the nucleus. Now, with the chopper cut the nucleus with a straight downward motion and then move the chopper to the left when you reach the center of the nucleus. In other words, your left hand moves the chopper like an inverted L. Do not go to the periphery for chopping but do it at the center. Once you have created a crack, split the nucleus till the center. Then rotate the nucleus 180 degrees and crack again so that you get two halves of the nucleus.

Now that you have two halves, you have a shelf to embed the probe. So, now place the probe with ultrasound into one half of the nucleus and chop. Like this create three quadrants in one half of the nucleus. Then make another three halves with the second half of the nucleus. Thus, you now have 6 quadrants or pie-shaped fragments.

Once all the pieces have been chopped, take out each piece one by one and in pulse phaco mode aspirate the pieces at the level of the iris. Do not work in the bag unless the cornea is preoperatively bad or the patient is very elderly.

The next step is to do cortical washing. Always try to remove the subincisional cortex first, as that is the most difficult. Note that everytime the left hand has the straight rod controlling the movements of the eye. If necessary use a bimanual irrigation aspiration technique. Then inject viscoelastic and implant the IOL. At the end of the procedure, inject the BSS inside the lips of the clear corneal incision. This will create a stromal hydration at the wound. This will create a whiteness, which will disappear after 4 to 5 hours. The advantage of this is that the wound gets sealed better.

Adverse Effects

- One is still not sure if extended contact of Trypan blue with the corneal endothelium produces corneal damage. At present, no cases have been reported as the Trypan blue is washed off with the viscoelastic and the BSS fluid.
- Postsurgical inflammatory reactions and some bullous keratopathy have been known to occur after using vital staining agents.
- Extreme care must be taken when using Trypan blue on patients who are hypersensitive to any of its components.
- During animal experiments, a teratogenic and/or mutagenic effect has been reported after repeated and/or high dose intraperitoneal or intravenous injections with Trypan blue. So, one should not use Trypan blue in pregnant women.

SUMMARY

Trypan blue can make life much easier for the phaco surgeon especially in cases of mature and hypermature cataracts by staining the anterior capsule. Another dye, is ICG, which is much costlier.

6

Small Pupil Phacoemulsification

Priya Narang, Amar Agarwal

INTRODUCTION

The pupil size has always played a very important role in performing any type of cataract surgery, be it an Intracapsular cataract extraction, extracapsular cataract extraction, phacoemulsification, bimanual phacoemulsification or microphakonit.

A large sized, well-dilated pupil increases the ease of surgery dramatically, but unfortunately a miotic pupil (less than 4.0 mm), is a common bugbear that every surgeon faces at some time or the other. Miotic, nondilating pupil (Fig. 6.1) may be secondary to a variety of reasons (Table 6.1). Phacoemulsification is especially difficult in these cases as it affects all steps right from capsulorhexis to emulsification of the nucleus, cortical removal and in-the-bag IOL insertion. The surgeon is forced to perform a small capsulorhexis, which further adds to the difficulty in performing surgery. A small pupil may cause damage to the patient's eye by emulsification of the iris or cause complications such as sphincter tears, intraoperative bleeding, zonular dialysis, posterior capsular rent or nucleus drop. Prolonged surgical time and increased maneuvering may result in

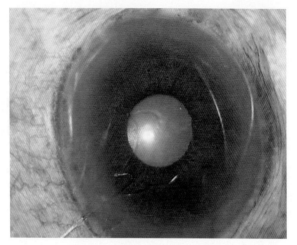

Figure 6.1 Miotic non-dilating pupil

TABLE 6.1 Causes for miotic pupil

- Age related dilator atrophy
- Diabetes mellitus
- Synechiae
- Previous trauma
- Previous surgery
- Uveitis
- Iridoschisis
- Pseudoexfoliation syndrome
- Chronic miotic therapy
- Congenital
- Idiopathic
- Marfan's syndrome
- Chronic lues

postoperative complications such as striate keratopathy, uveitis, secondary glaucoma, floppy, torn or atrophic iris, irregular pupil, endophthalmitis, cystoid macular edema, etc. all resulting in a suboptimal surgical outcome and an unhappy patient. A study of 1,000 consecutive extracapsular cataract extractions showed that a small pupil was the most common factor associated with vitreous loss and capsular rupture.[1]

A hypotonic, mid-dilated, irregular pupil postoperatively can also be aesthetically bad, especially noticeable in light colored irides. Such a pupil can also have significant effect on the pupillary function leading onto iatrogenic glare dysfunction. Masket reported that an enlarged pupil can be responsible for postoperative glare disability in eyes that were anatomically normal except for having pseudophakia.[2] All these factors makes it mandatory, especially for a phaco surgeon to know how to tackle a miotic pupil.

There are a variety of techniques for the management of the small pupil, including iris hooks, iris rings, and pupillary stretching with or without the use of multiple half-width sphincterotomies.[3]

PREOPERATIVE EVALUATION

A dilated preoperative examination is mandatory for every patient, not just for assessing the posterior segment, but also to detect cases of suboptimal pupillary dilatation. Appropriate history is important for detecting any underlying etiology for the miotic pupil. One should check for intraoperative floppy iris syndrome and usage of tamsulosin (Flomax®, Boehringer-Ingelheim Pharmaceuticals, Inc., Ridgefield, CT) as suggested by David Chang. A careful slit lamp examination is mandatory for detecting the cause as well as any associated complicating conditions that may co-exist, such as zonular weakness in a case of pseudoexfoliation. Proper planning of the surgical steps should be done preoperatively itself. Synechiolysis or membranectomy may be required in cases of chronic uveitis. For patients on chronic miotic therapy, these drugs should stopped preoperatively and replaced if necessary with other suitable medications.

PHARMACOLOGICAL MYDRIASIS

The topical agents used preoperatively for dilating the patient's eye should include a cycloplegic, a mydriatic and a nonsteroidal anti-inflammatory drug.[4]

Cycloplegics

The most commonly used cycloplegic agent is cyclopentolate hydrochloride 1%, which provides good cycloplegia and pupillary dilatation. The pupillary dilatation can last up to 36 hours. Tropicamide hydrochloride 1% is also a good pupillary dilator though shorter acting and with slightly lesser degree of cycloplegia. Atropine sulfate 1% is a longer lasting mydriatic and can be considered in cases of chronic uveitis, long-standing diabetics, etc.

Mydriatics

Phenylephrine hydrochloride 2.5%, is a good pupil dilator, especially when combined with a cycloplegic. The 10% solution gives stronger dilatation, especially in resistant cases but the disadvantage is that it may increase the blood pressure in some patients and can also result in corneal punctate keratopathy. Mydricaine, a product which contains atropine, procaine and adrenaline can also be used as sub-conjunctival injections preoperatively.

NSAIDs

Nonsteroidal anti-inflammatory drugs decrease the incidence of intraoperative constriction of the pupil. This is especially important in case of prolonged surgeries and surgery with increased intra-operative manipulation. Suprofen, diclofenac ketorolac, flurbiprofen, etc. are commonly used for this purpose.[5-10]

TABLE 6.2 Methods for enlarging the pupil

- Sphincter sparing techniques:
  - Synechiolysis
  - Pupillary membranectomy
  - Viscomydriasis
- Sphincter involving techniques:
  - Mini sphincterotomies
  - Pupil stretch
  - Iris hooks
  - Pupil ring expanders

Pharmacological mydriasis may not be effective in all cases, especially in cases with posterior synechiae and scarred pupils. Such pupils have to be dealt with appropriately during surgery to avoid a cascade of complications (Table 6.2).

Intraoperative Procedures not Involving the Sphincter

Viscomydriasis

A new ophthalmic viscosurgical device (OVD), 2.4% Hyaluronate can be used for mechanically dilating the pupil in certain cases.[4,11] It is injected into the center of the pupil to mechanically dissect any synechiae and to stretch the sphincter. It should be completely removed at the end of the procedure to avoid postoperative intraocular pressure increase.

Synechiolysis

A blunt spatula is passed through the sideport incision after injecting viscoelastic into the eye.[4] A second side port incision may be required in case of extensive synechiae. This is followed by utilizing one of the other techniques to maintain the pupil in a dilated stage, e.g. viscomydriasis, iris hooks, pupil expanders, etc. A blunt rod can also be used to sweep any posterior synechiae free, without any stretch motions (Fig. 6.2).

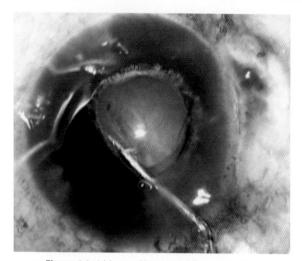

Figure 6.2 A blunt rod being used for synechiolysis

Pupillary Membranectomy

Pupillary membranes can cause small pupils. These membranes can be then care of with a combination of preoperative pharmacotherapy and intraoperative surgical removal by stripping the fine fibrin pupillary membrane using Utrata forceps.

Intraoperative Procedures Involving the Sphincter

Mini Sphincterotomies

Mini sphincterotomies[4,11] can be done with either vannas scissors through the main port incision or with vitreoretinal scissors placed through the paracentesis. Very small partial cuts, no larger than 0.75 mm in radial length, are made limited to the sphincter tissue. As long as the incisions are kept very small, postoperatively the pupil should be normal both functionally and esthetically. The disadvantage is that regardless of the wound position, the incision is more difficult to create in the clock hour of the wound.

Pupil Stretch

Pupil stretch[12] can be done either using push-pull instruments or pronged instruments which stretch the pupillary sphincter. Pupillary stretching generally causes multiple fine partial sphincter tears. If combined with preplaced mini-sphincterotomies, the effect can be increased.[3] It generally results in a functionally and esthetically acceptable pupil postoperatively. The disadvantage is that the iris sometimes becomes flaccid and may either move into an undesirable location or may prolapse through the incision during surgery. Rarely, it may cause complications like hematoma or larger sphincter tears, pigment dispersion, postoperative uveitis, pressure spike and an abnormal and nonfunctional pupil postoperatively.

Bimanual Push-pull Instruments

Using viscoelastic cover, two hooks are used in a slow, controlled fashion, to stretch the pupil in one or more axes.[2] One hook is used for pushing the pupillary margin and the other one for pulling. The push-pull should be done simultaneously, in a controlled manner, to avoid large sphincter tears. This technique usually achieves an adequately sized pupil for effective phacoemulsification. A two-handed, two-instrument bimanual stretch technique with an angled Kuglen hook and Lindstrom star nucleus rotator is very effective.

Pronged Instruments

Instruments available[12] are the Keuch two-pronged pupil stretcher (Katena) or the four-pronged pupil stretcher (Rhein Medical's Beehler pupil dilator). Postoperatively, the pupil continues to react normally. This technique, popularized by Luther Fry[4] is an efficient and cost-effective method. The prongs (Fig. 6.3) should be maintained parallel to the iris plane and should not slip out into

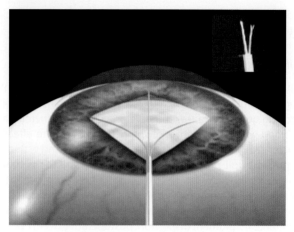

Figure 6.3 Tri-pronged pupil stretchers

the pupil margin, especially on starting to depress the plunger to create the pupil stretch.

Iris Hooks

Commercially available iris hooks (Grieshaber, Schaffhausen, Switzerland) have been originally used for posterior segment surgeries.[13] They can also be utilized for phacoemulsification[14] (Figs 6.4 to 6.6), but the disadvantage is that unless properly placed, they can pull the iris diaphragm forwards, resulting in chaffing and thermal damage during phacoemulsification.[15,16] To avoid this, the hooks should be placed parallel to the iris plane through small, short tract, peripheral paracenteses or by releasing the hooks after creating the capsulorhexis but before phacoemulsification. Gradual enlargement of the pupil should be done and one a pupil size just enough for the surgical procedure should be attempted for to avoid postoperative pupillary atony. The other disadvantage is that it adds to the time and cost of surgery. Iris hooks have also been used in

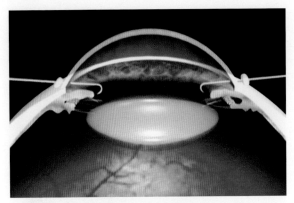

Figure 6.4 Iris hooks inserted to enlarge the pupil

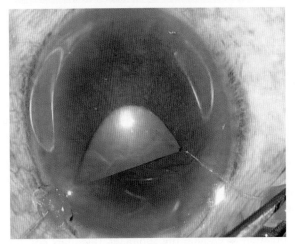

Figure 6.5 Iris hooks being placed

cases of zonular dialysis to stabilize the capsular bag by hooking it around the capsulorhexis margin.

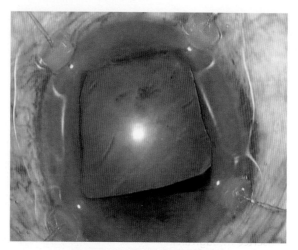

Figure 6.6 All four iris hooks in place

IRIS RETAINER METHODS

Pupil Ring Expanders

They enlarge the pupil without sphincter damage. Here, incomplete pupil ring expanders are used to stretch the pupil.[17] They are inserted through the main port and manipulated into the pupil space. They can create the largest diameter pupil, creating a uniform expanding force around approximately 300° of the pupil. They thus have the least tendency for sphincter tears, as they do not produce point pressure on the pupillary margin. The disadvantages with these devices are that they are rigid, cumbersome and slightly difficult to insert into the eye through a small incision. They require manipulation to engage the sphincter. They may also hamper entry, exit and maneuvering of additional instruments through the incisions. It also adds to the time and cost of surgery. The one-piece retaining rings are often difficult to position and even more difficult to remove.

Three expanders are the Grather, Siepser and Morcher[4] (Table 6.2). They are made of solid PMMA, silicone, or expansible hydrogel material.

The Graether's pupil expander consists of a silicone ring with an indentation, which fits all along the edge of the pupil.[18] The iris fits like a tyre around the ring which is like an iron wheel. The disadvantage is that it can loosen easily with intraocular maneuvers.

Perfect Pupil Device™

Developed by John Milverton, MD of Sydney, Australia, it is a sterile, disposable, flexible polyurethane ring with an integrated arm (Fig. 6.7) that allows for easy insertion and removal.[11] It is inserted with a forceps or injected with an injector through the main port. The integrated arm remains outside the eye to aid in easy removal. It can be inserted through an incision less than 100 microns. Because of the open ring design of the Perfect Pupil™, there is no interference with other instrumentation.

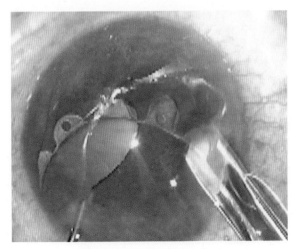

Figure 6.7 Perfect pupil device

Use of Malyugin Ring for Small Pupil Phacoemulsification

The Malyugin ring (Fig. 6.8) is a new device which has proved itself very useful for safe phacoemulsification in eyes with small, non-dilating pupils. The Malyugin ring is a square shaped, transitory implant with four circular scrolls that hold the iris at equidistant points with a gentle, stretching force. Insertion of the ring generally results in a pupillary diameter of about 6 mm, adequate for most phaco procedures. It keeps the iris sphincter from getting damaged during phaco procedures and allows the pupil to return to its normal size, shape and function at the end of surgery.

It has multiple advantages over the iris hooks. It is easier to implant and doesn't need multiple paracenteses wounds for insertion as it is introduced through the main port incision. Operating time is reduced and all risks associated with increased number of incisions are eliminated. It has no pointed ends and acts by producing a gentle, expansile force distributed over a wider area of contact with the pupil, thus causing lesser iris trauma. It may be especially useful in intraoperative floppy iris (IFIS) syndrome as there

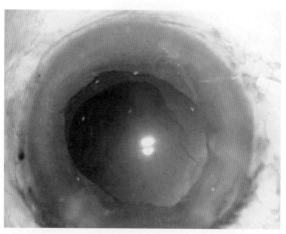

Figure 6.8 Malyugin ring

is lesser chances of iris prolapse as may occur in case of iris hooks through incorrectly sized paracenteses.

Modified Malyugin Ring Iris Expansion Technique in Small-Pupil Cataract Surgery with Posterior Capsule Defect

Agarwal et al. modified the technique (Fig. 6.9) for using the Malyugin ring for safe iris expansion in small-pupil cataract surgery in eyes with posterior capsule defects. This modification has 2 main advantages. First, while the ring is being injected, the chances of it dropping into the vitreous due to poor capsule support is reduced as it is well secured by the suture. Second, if a large posterior capsule defect occurs and the ring slips into the vitreous, it can be pulled back easily with the suture end. Thus, the surgeon can work effectively below the pupillary plane without fear of the ring slipping into the vitreous.

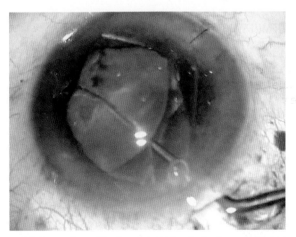

Figure 6.9 Agarwal's modification of the Malyugin ring in eyes with posterior capsular rupture

Surgical Complications

Bleeding may occur with these techniques.[4] It generally subsides on its own and any postoperative hyphema gets absorbed spontaneously. In case of significant bleeding intraoperatively, the intraocular pressure should be increased by elevating the bottle height, or by injecting a viscoelastic agent or air to the eye. In case of a major, unresponsive bleed within the eye, one can add fibrin. Instrument-related damages that can occur include corneal endothelial damage,[4] iridodialysis, bleeding, iris pigment dispersion, etc. Postoperatively, the patient may have an atonic, distorted pupil. Large tears to the iris sphincter can result in this. Pupillary dilatation should be done gradually to minimize sphincter tears and only the minimum amount of stretching that is required for the surgical steps should be done.[4] A forcibly, maximally dilated pupil can result in postoperative atonic pupil. Other postoperative complications which can be seen include uveitis, increased intraocular pressure, pigments on the IOL, etc. These can be avoided by careful, gentle instrumentation and as less manipulation as possible within the eye.

PHACOEMULSIFICATION PEARLS

- The experience of the surgeon and the nature of the cataract dictate the minimum pupil diameter for a case.
- Generally, if the pupil is large enough to perform an adequate capsulorhexis, it is large enough for the remainder of the surgical procedure.
- In cases with small pupil, the corneal incision must be made anteriorly to avoid the risk of iris prolapse with posterior corneal incisions.
- Capsular dyes such as indocyanine green (ICG) or trypan blue should be injected under the iris to aid in making the rhexis as well as to visualize the capsule as the pupil later enlarges.
- Hydrodissection should be gentle as an excessive fluid wave can cause iris prolapse.

- A retentive viscoelastic such as Healon5 should be used as it pressurizes the anterior chamber. As the intraocular pressure (IOP) increases, the viscoelastic remains in the eye and pushes down on the lens-iris diaphragm, thus mechanically enlarging the pupil. A cohesive type of viscoelastic is not as effective as it evacuates easily from the eye when IOP increases.
- Mini-sphincterotomies or the bimanual stretching technique of Luther Fry work well with fibrotic pupils such as those in patients on chronic miotic therapy. They are not as effective when the iris is elastic and floppy because the sphincter does not readily tear and the iris snaps back following stretching.
- A Sinskey or Kuglen hook can be inserted through the sideport incision to move the pupil away while doing capsulorhexis to achieve a larger sized rhexis.
- Sculpting is more difficult with small pupils as visualization is poor. The peripheral lens cannot be seen and the red reflex, which is required to visualize the depth of sculpting, is reduced by the smaller pupil diameter. These problems are overcome to a large extent using phaco chop techniques.
- For nucleus removal phaco chop, particularly vertical chop is the ideal technique in a miotic pupil, as it does not require a large pupil. Here, the phaco tip stays in the center of the pupil for the majority of the time, and the chances of capturing the iris or capsular edge is much lesser. The second instrument can be used to move the pupil away to get a perfect position and then phaco chop can be performed.
- An injector is preferred over the folding forceps for inserting the IOL. The tip of the folder may catch the iris in the presence of iris prolapse or a flaccid iris and cause a dialysis. The injector tip immediately plugs the incision and there will be a net influx of viscoelastic instead.
- An injector separates the IOL from the surrounding tissues keeping it sterile. It also helps in exact positioning of the IOL which is an advantage in a small pupil or a flaccid iris.

- As long as the tip of the injector fits into the capsulorhexis, the IOL can be delivered into the bag without stretching or tearing the capsulorhexis.
- The second instrument or viscoelastic can be used to push the iris back and away from the bevel of the injector where it might otherwise be caught.
- For the trailing haptic, two instruments can be used — one to hold the iris and the other to dial in the trailing haptic.
- With plate haptic IOLs, anterior capsular contracture is greater and there is also more giant cell reaction, hence older silicone IOLs should be avoided in eyes that are likely to be inflamed.
- Latest generation silicone IOLs, such as Clariflex (AMO), have no difference in long-term inflammatory profiles between hydrophobic acrylic and second generation silicone. The latest generation silicone achieved statistically significantly less inflammation than the AcrySof IOL in the long-term. The second- and higher-generation silicone IOLs are also more chemically pure and have a better overall design with a higher refractive index and thinner profile. Silicone IOLs also have a greater ease of implantation and reduced incision size as compared to acrylic IOLs.
- The Unfolder Emerald injector allows the surgeon to use a full size 6-mm optic acrylic IOL in a three-piece model through a 3-mm incision.
- A Lester hook (Katena Products, Inc.) can be used in the second hand to retract the pupil to re-tear and enlarge a small capsulorhexis.
- Irrespective of the method chosen for enlarging the pupil during phacoemulsification, the pupil should be constricted at the end of surgery with an intraocular miotic. If necessary, the pupil should be stroked with a blunt, gentle instrument to reduce its size. This prevents optic capture, capsular adhesion or other manner of pupillary deformity.

- Postoperatively, topical anti-inflammatory agents should be used to take care of the increased inflammatory activity secondary to increased maneuvering and longer and more difficult surgery.

REFERENCES

1. Guzek JP, Holm M, Cotter JB, et al. Risk factors for intraoperative complications in 1000 extracapsular cataract cases. Ophthalmology. 1987;94:46-466.
2. Masket S. Relationship between postoperative pupil. In: size and disability glare. J Cataract Refract Surg. 1992;(18):506-7.
3. Fine IH: Phacoemulsification in the presence of a small pupil. In: Steinert RF (ed). Cataract Surgery: Technique, Complications and Management. Philadelphia, PA, WB Saunders. 1995.pp.199-208.
4. Masket S. Cataract surgery complicated by the miotic pupil. In: Buratto L, Osher RH, Masket S, (eds). Cataract Surgery in Complicated Cases. Thorofare, NJ: Slack. 2000.pp.131-7.
5. Thaller VT, Kulshrestha MK, Bell K. The effect of pre-operative topical flurbiprofen or diclofenac on pupil dilatation. Eye. 2000;14(Pt4):642-5.
6. Snyder RW, Siekert RW, Schwiegerling J, Donnenfeld E, Thompson P. Acular as a single agent for use as an antimiotic and anti-inflammatory in cataract surgery. J Cataract Refract Surg. 2000;26(8):1225-7.
7. Gupta VP, Dhaliwal U, Prasad N. Ketorolac tromethamine in the maintenance of intraoperative mydriasis. Ophthalmic Surg Lasers. 1997;28(9):731-8.
8. Solomon KD, Turkalj JW, Whiteside SB, Stewart JA, Apple DJ. Topical 0.5% ketorolac vs 0.03% flurbiprofen for inhibition of miosis during cataract surgery. Arch Ophthalmol. 1997;115(9):1119-22.
9. Gimbel H, Van Westenbrugge J, Cheetham JK, DeGryse R, Garcia CG. Intraocular availability and pupillary effect of flurbiprofen and indomethacin during cataract surgery. J Cataract Refract Surg. 1996;22(4):474-9.
10. Brown RM, Roberts CW. Preoperative and postoperative use of nonsteroidal antiinflammatory drugs in cataract surgery. Insight. 1996;21(1):13-6.
11. Kershner, RM. "Management of the Small Pupil in Clear Corneal Cataract Surgery." J Cataract Refract Surg. 2002;28.

12. Shephard DM. The pupil stretch technique for miotic pupils in cataract surgery. Ophthalmic Surg. 1994;24:851-2.
13. De Juan Jr E, Hickingbotham D. Flexible iris retractors. Am J Ophthalmol. 1991;111:766-7.
14. Smith GT, Liu CSC. Flexible iris hooks for phacoemulsification in patients with iridoschisis. J Cataract Refract Surg. 2000;26:1277-80.
15. Nichamin LD. Enlarging the pupil for cataract extraction using flexible nylon iris retractors. J Cataract Refract Surg. 1993:19:793-6.
16. Masket S. Avoiding complications associated with iris retractor use in small pupil cataract extraction. J Cataract Refract Surg. 1996;22:168-71.
17. Graether JM. Graether pupil expander for managing the small pupil during surgery. J Cataract Refract Surg. 1996;22:530-5.
18. Benjamin Boyd. Phacoemulsification in small pupils. In: The Art and Science of Cataract Surgery; Highlights of Ophthalmology. 2001.

Combined Cataract and Glaucoma Surgery

Amar Agarwal, Priya Narang

INTRODUCTION

Cataract is the foremost cause of blindness worldwide and continues to remain an important cause of visual impairment in the United States.[1-4] In the Baltimore Eye Survey, cataract was found to be the leading cause of blindness among the population over 40 years of age, and unoperated cataract was found to be four times more common among African Americans than Caucasian Americans.[3] The Salisbury Eye Evaluation Study (n=2,520) found that after refractive error, cataract was the leading cause of visual impairment in African Americans and Caucasian Americans.[4]

Cataract and glaucoma often co-exist in the elderly, especially so with the increasing longevity of the human race. It is especially important to be able to appropriately manage this patient sub-group in whom central vision is compromised due to cataract and peripheral vision due to the glaucoma.

SURGICAL OPTIONS

When a patient with cataract also has glaucoma, surgical options are cataract surgery alone, glaucoma surgery first followed later by cataract surgery, cataract surgery first followed later by glaucoma surgery, or cataract surgery combined with filtering surgery. The decision is based on the degree of visual field damage, optic nerve head damage and retinal nerve fibre layer loss, the patient's response to medical or laser therapy, grade of cataract, and the surgeon's experience and personal preferences. The factors favoring a combined procedure are many. While cataract surgery with IOL implantation lowers IOP by 2 to 4 mm Hg in long-term studies,[5,6] a glaucoma procedure combined with cataract surgery lowers IOP more effectively (6–8 mm Hg).[7-9] Following either extracapsular cataract extraction (ECCE) or phacoemulsification, many of the glaucomatous eyes suffer an IOP spike to 30 mm Hg or more, which may lead onto anterior ischemic optic neuropathy or progressive glaucomatous damage. It is essential to avoid IOP spikes in eyes with severe optic disc damage and visual field loss close to fixation. Combining drainage surgery with cataract extraction can significantly reduce the frequency of these spikes. The disadvantages for performing filtration surgery first followed by cataract surgery 3 to 6 months after a mature bleb has formed include delayed visual recovery, all attendant anesthetic as well as perioperative risks of having to undergo two intraocular surgical procedures, decreased cost efficiency and the possibility of inducing bleb failure.

In a patient who requires both cataract extraction and glaucoma surgery for IOP control, a combined surgery would be preferred. The advantages of a combined procedure (cataract extraction with IOL implantation and trabeculectomy) are avoiding the IOP rise that may occur following cataract surgery alone, rapid visual recovery, and long-term glaucoma control with a single operation. Phacoemulsification combined with trabeculectomy results in good IOP control as well as an improvement in the visual acuity.[7,10,11] The disadvantage of combined procedures is that they are technically slightly more difficult and time consuming.

In a patient for whom only glaucoma surgery is definitely indicated, the decision to combine it with a cataract extraction as well depends on the patient's age, visual acuity, visual requirements, grade of cataract, associated ocular comorbidity such as subluxated lens, pseudoexfoliation syndrome, etc. Trabeculectomy hastens the onset and progression of cataract which will make optic nerve head and field evaluation difficult and also result in an unhappy patient who then requires a second surgery for the cataract soon after. The second step cataract surgery may also result in failure of a previously functioning bleb, all of which lead to an extremely unhappy patient and a difficult situation for the surgeon. All these factors favor a combined surgery for these patients.[12]

One may also consider combining glaucoma surgery in a patient who is going to undergo a cataract extraction depending on the IOP control, number of drugs required for IOP control and patient's intolerance or non-compliance with drugs.[12]

PREOPERATIVE PREPARATION

Apart from the usual preoperative preparations, it is extremely imperative to control the IOP prior to surgery to avoid choroidal effusion, choroidal hemorrhage or expulsive hemorrhage. Phacoemulsification is especially advantageous here, as it is a closed chamber procedure, nevertheless, IOP may suddenly drop to values close to zero even with phaco.[13] Preoperative control of IOP can be done with topical medications, systemic carbonic anhydrase inhibitors, oral glycerol or intravenous mannitol.

SURGICAL TECHNIQUES

Peripheral Iridectomy with Phacoemulsification

A simple peripheral iridectomy can be done with a vitrectomy probe at the time of phacoemulsification in some cases of angle closure glaucoma. Care should be taken that the iridectomy is in a position that is covered by the lids in order to avoid intractable monocular diplopia for the patient.

Single Site Trabeculectomy with Phacoemulsification

Either a limbus based or fornix based conjunctival flap is created followed by a scleral flap which will be large enough to allow implantation of the IOL (Fig. 7.1). Anterior chamber is entered under the scleral flap and phacoemulsification is performed as usual. After IOL implantation, sclerectomy and iridectomy are made and the scleral and conjunctival flaps are sutured.

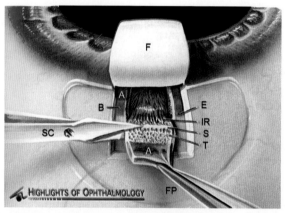

Figure 7.1 Trabeculectomy with Fornix Based Flap—removing the trabecular window—surgeon's view. This is a surgeon's view of the final incision to remove the trabecular window. It also reveals the surgeon's view of the structures most important to proper trabeculectomy. The trabeculectomy flap which is being excised has been hinged backwards exposing its deep surface to the surgeon's view. The Vannas scissors (SC), make the final cut just in front of the scleral spur (S), on the trabecular tissue which is here being reflected back with forceps (FP). The scleral spur is localized externally (E) by the junction of white sclera and gray band (B). Scleral flap (F). Clear cornea (A). Iris (I). Iris root (IR). Trabeculum (T).

(*Courtesy:* Highlights of Ophthalmology, "Innovations in the glaucomas: etiology, diagnosis and management", English edition, 2002. Editors: Benjamin F Boyd, MD, FACS; Maurice H Luntz, MD, FACS; Co-editor: Samuel Boyd, MD)

Two Site Trabeculectomy with Phacoemulsification

Conjunctival and scleral flaps are made at the beginning of the surgery. Clear corneal phacoemulsification is then carried out in another quadrant. Filtering surgery is then completed at the end of the surgery (Figs 7.2 A and B).

Trabeculectomy with Microphakonit

Here 0.7 mm gauge phaco probe, irrigating chopper and irrigation/aspiration (I/A) instruments are used for performing bimanual micro incision cataract surgery. Trabeculectomy is performed as previously mentioned (Figs 7.3 A to C).

Trabeculotomy with Phacoemulsification, Single Site and Two Site

In trabeculotomy,[14] a direct communication is created between the anterior chamber and the Schlemm's canal (Fig. 7.1). The

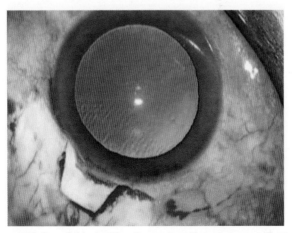

Figure 7.2A Superficial scleral flap dissected out. Then phacoemulsification is done in another site and the IOL implanted

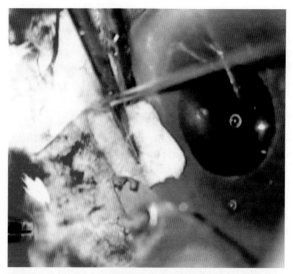

Figure 7.2B Inner scleral window about to be made after IOL insertion

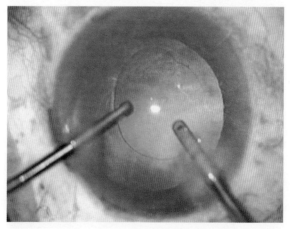

Figure 7.3A Microphakonit being performed using 0.7 mm gauge instruments after making superficial scleral flap. Cortex has been removed with 0.7 mm gauge instruments in microphakonit

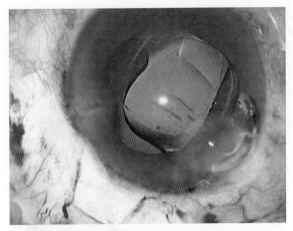

Figure 7.3B IOL inserted after enlarging the microphakonit incision

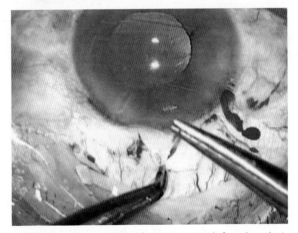

Figure 7.3C The superficial scleral flap being sutured after taking the inner scleral punch and performing the iridectomy

conjunctival and scleral flaps are raised. In single site surgery, the scleral flap is then incised from its backside with a shallow incision, from which a sclero-corneal pocket is dissected with a keratome for the phaco probe. In two site surgery, the phacoemulsification is done from a different quadrant. Next, the Schlemm's canal is identified by its pigmentation and by the blood refluxed into the canal during phacoemulsification. In case of difficulty in identification because of too thick a remaining scleral bed, a second inner scleral flap is raised. Once the overlying sclera is thick enough, the Schlemm's canal can be easily identified. The scleral lamellae over Schlemm's canal are then incised parallel to the canal taking care to avoid entering the anterior chamber. This can be facilitated by lifting the incised roof of Schlemm's canal with a fine forceps and widening the incision after an initial puncture in the roof with fine Vannas scissors. A specially curved canalicular probe is then inserted into the Schlemm's canal, and the trabecular meshwork ruptured with a forward and inward motion. This is then repeated on the opposite side as well through the same entry site. The scleral flap and conjunctiva are closed in a water tight manner.

NONPENETRATING GLAUCOMA SURGERY WITH PHACOEMULSIFICATION

Viscocanalostomy and Phacoemulsification

It is a nonperforating technique described by Stegman in 1991. It is aimed at avoiding fibrosis related bleb failure. It works by facilitating outflow of aqueous through the physiological pathway, viz. canal of Schlemm and the collector channels. This is done by creating a Descemetic window which is composed of the innermost layers of the trabecular meshwork and the Descemet's membrane.[15] Aqueous flows out through these layers and collects in an intrascleral space, through which it flows into the cut ends of the Schlemm's canal, which has been dilated previously by injecting high viscosity viscoelastic. It has also been postulated that there may be increased uveoscleral outflow after the surgery. The advantages of viscocanalostomy are that as it is a nonpenetrating procedure, postoperative complications such as hypotony, shallow anterior chamber, uveitis, endophthalmitis and cataract formation are avoided. Also the lack of external filtration avoids all bleb related complications such as bleb failure due to scarring, blebitis, discomfort, etc.

Under retrobulbar or peribulbar anesthesia, a fornix-based conjunctival flap is made. As little cautery as possible is used to avoid damage to Schlemm's canal and the collector channels. An outer parabolic flap, sized 5 × 5 mm, approximately 200 μm thick, is then dissected, followed by an inner 4 × 4 mm scleral flap. One should be able to see the dark reflex from the underlying choroid after dissecting the inner flap. The cut is advanced towards the limbus and the Schlemm's canal is deroofed. The two openings of the canal remain patent at the lateral edges of the cut. The inner flap is then extended into the clear cornea by approximately 1 mm using blunt dissection with a cotton tipped applicator. The inner scleral flap is then excised and the ostia of Schlemm's canal are cannulated with a specific cannula through which high-molecular-weight sodium hyaluronate (Healon GV®, Pharmacia & Upjohn, Sweden) is injected to distend it. This is done to prevent collapse and scarring in the early postoperative period. If adequate percolation is not seen through the Descemetic window, the juxtacanalicular meshwork along with the inner wall of the Schlemm's canal can be stripped with a fine forceps. The outer scleral flap is then tightly sutured and Healon GV® is injected beneath the flap to prevent the intrascleral lake from collapsing and scarring in the early postoperative period. Two lateral stitches hold the conjunctiva in place. The conjunctiva is then closed. In case of perforation of the Descemetic window, one can convert to a trabeculectomy. Viscocanalostomy can be combined with phacoemulsification[15] using the same site or a different site. In single site, phacoemulsification is done via a superior scleral tunnel and a block of deep sclera is excised at the end and viscocanalostomy is completed as usual. In case of two site surgery, viscocanalostomy is done after phaco has been completed through the temporal approach. When viscocanalostomy is combined with phaco, aqueous leakage from the tunnel can be differentiated from a perforation of the Descemetic membrane by drying the window surface with a sponge.

Deep Sclerectomy and Phacoemulsification

It is also a non-penetrating surgery, which differs from viscocanalostomy by producing sub-Tenon filtration.

Under retrobulbar or peribulbar anesthesia, a 4 × 4 mm, 200 to 250 microns square superficial scleral flap is made followed by a deep scleral flap similar to that in viscocanalostomy. The dissection is extended anteriorly to deroof the Schlemm's canal and a Descemetic window is created. The deep flap is excised and the superficial flap is closed less tightly to allow percolation into the sub-Tenon space. The conjunctiva is then closed.[15]

Collagen or reticulated hyaluronic acid implants[15] can be inserted into the scleral lake for improving long-term filtration. These devices are slowly absorbed, thus maintaining the intrascleral lake and preventing its closure by fibrosis. A high molecular weight viscoelastic[15] (Healon5) may also be injected into the intrascleral lake to decrease wound healing. Deep sclerectomy can also be combined with the application of antimetabolites.[15] The hypotensive effect may also be increased even after surgery by perforating the Descemetic window ab interno with a YAG laser.

Deep sclerectomy can be combined with phacoemulsification just as in viscocanalostomy.

Laser Sclerotomy with Phacoemulsification

Here, the laser fiberoptic of the Nd YAG laser is passed through the clear corneal incision and a short burst of laser is given directly opposite the planned site of sclerotomy.[16] The aiming beam is used as a guide and hence a goniolens is not required. When the aiming beam is seen around 1.5 mm from the limbus, a short burst of laser brings the laser fiberoptic out of the sclera and under the conjunctiva. The laser fiberoptic has a Helium Neon aiming beam and the diameter of the optic end is 380 microns. The fiberoptic is encased in a silicone sleeve. The remaining phacoemulsification is carried out as usual.

Seton Procedure

This can be done in cases which do not respond to conventional surgeries (Fig. 7.4).

Antimetabolites

The use of antifibrotics (mitomycin-C,[17] and 5-fluorouracil[18] to reduce the potential for bleb failure in combined phacotrabeculectomy is controversial. Mitomycin-C may result in lower long-term IOPs when used with combined procedures[9,17] but 5-fluorouracil does not seem to.[9,18] The potential vision-threatening complications of antimetabolites such as bleb-related endophthalmitis[19,20] hypotonic maculopathy[21,22] and late-onset bleb leaks[23] should be considered while deciding to use these agents.

Type of IOL

Friedrich et al. found that foldable silcone IOLs may induce late postoperative inflammatory membranes with pigment precipitates, especially after combined surgery.[24]

COMPLICATIONS

Postoperative uveitis or rise in IOP can usually be tackled with appropriate medications. Hyphema, if small usually resolves by itself. If very large, it may need to be evacuated. Excessive filtration may occur leading onto choroidal detachment. When associated with a flat anterior chamber or other severe complications, it may require fluid drainage and bleb revision. Shallow anterior chamber may also be due to bleb leak. Hypotonic maculopathy may rarely be seen, especially in a young myopic patient. Other postoperative complications which may occur after routine phacoemulsification

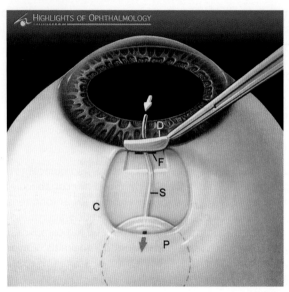

Figure 7.4 Seton implantation procedure: A fornix based conjunctival flap (C) is raised and the methyl methacrylate baseplate (P) of the Seton is pushed under the conjunctival flap posteriorly and sutured to the scleral surface. The implant has a biconcave shape with the inferior surface shaped to fit the sclera. A small 3 mm square half thickness lamellar scleral flap (D) is raised just as in a trabeculectomy. An incision (F) is made into the anterior chamber under this scleral flap and the long silicone tube (S) of the Seton is placed into the anterior chamber (the end of the silicone tube can be seen in the anterior chamber near the tip of the white arrow). Next, the scleral flap (D) is sutured down around the tube (S) of the Seton. Finally, the conjunctiva is sutured back in place. Aqueous then drains from the anterior chamber (white arrow) down through the tube (S) to the baseplate (P) (black arrow), where a bleb forms.

(*Courtesy:* Highlights of Ophthalmology, "Innovations in the glaucomas: etiology, diagnosis and management", English edition, 2002. Editors: Benjamin F Boyd, MD, FACS; Maurice H Luntz, MD, FACS; Co-editor: Samuel Boyd, MD)

may occur in this setting too. Late postoperative complications include cystoid macular edema, capsular phimosis syndrome, IOL decentration, posterior capsular opacification, bleb failure, bleb related endophthalmitis, etc.

Key Points

- The summary of the evidence on intraocular pressure control with surgical treatment of coexisting cataract and glaucoma on long-term intraocular pressure control[25] states that there is good evidence that long-term IOP control is greater with combined procedures than with cataract extraction alone and fair evidence that trabeculectomy alone lowers long-term IOP more than combined ECCE and trabeculectomy. There is weak evidence that cataract extraction in glaucoma patients lowers IOP on average by 2 to 4 mm Hg, trabeculectomy alone appears to lower IOP more than combined phaco and trabeculectomy, phaco and trabeculectomy lowers IOP by approximately 8 mm Hg in individuals followed up for a mean of 1 to 2 years, ECCE and trabeculectomy lowers IOP by approximately 6 to 8 mm Hg in individuals followed up for a mean of 1 to 2 years. The evidence was insufficient to determine the impact of cataract extraction on preexisting filtering blebs, to determine if other combined techniques (e.g., cyclodialysis and endolaser) work as well as cataract extraction and trabeculectomy and to determine if combined phaco and trabeculectomy lowers IOP on the first postoperative day more than phaco alone.
- An evidence-based practice center sponsored by the Agency for Healthcare Research and Quality reviewed 131 studies on the treatment of adults with coexisting cataract and glaucoma, assessed the study quality and data, and reported it in evidence tables.[9] The investigators concluded that the findings that glaucoma surgery was associated with an increased risk of postoperative cataract and that a glaucoma procedure added to cataract surgery lowers IOP more than cataract surgery alone were strongly supported by the literature.
- The other findings that were found to be moderately supported by the literature[9] were that limbus- and fornix-based conjunctival incisions provided the same degree of long-term IOP lowering in combined surgery; in combined surgery using phacoemulsification, the size of the cataract incision did not affect long-term IOP control; when used with combined procedures 5-fluorouracil was not beneficial in further lowering IOP whereas mitomycin-C was efficacious in producing lower long-term IOPs when used with combined procedures.

Contd...

Contd...

- Findings weakly supported by literature[9] are that combined procedures resulted in lower IOP at 24 hours than cataract extraction alone; extracapsular cataract extraction (ECCE) alone appears to increase IOP at 24 hours; in the long term, cataract surgery alone lowered IOP by 2 to 4 mm Hg, combined cataract and glaucoma surgery lowered IOP by 6 to 8 mm Hg, and the performance of a glaucoma procedure alone provided even greater long-term IOP lowering than combined cataract and glaucoma surgery; combined surgery in which the incisions for the cataract extraction and glaucoma procedure are separate provided slightly lower long-term IOP than a one-site approach and that combined surgery in which phacoemulsification is used provided slightly lower long-term IOP than nuclear expression.
- It is extremely imperative to control the IOP prior to surgery to avoid choroidal effusion, choroidal hemorrhage or expulsive hemorrhage.
- Newer techniques combining non-penetrating glaucoma surgery with phacoemulsification appear promising but long-term follow-up results have to be reported before they become widely practised.

REFERENCES

1. Age-related Eye Disease Study Research Group. A randomized, placebo-controlled clinical trial of high-dose supplementation with vitamins C and E and beta carotene for age-related cataract and vision loss: AREDS Report No. 9. Arch Ophthalmol. 2001;119:1439-52.
2. Sperduto RD, Hu TS, Milton RC, et al. The Linxian cataract studies. Two nutrition intervention trials. Arch Ophthalmol. 1993;111:1246-53.
3. Mares-Perlman JA, Klein BE, Klein R, Ritter LL. Relation between lens opacities and vitamin and mineral supplement use. Ophthalmology. 1994;101:315-25.
4. Leske MC, Wu SY, Connell AM, et al. Lens opacities, demographic factors and nutritional supplements in the Barbados Eye Study. Int J Epidemiol. 1997;26:1314-22.
5. Shingleton BJ, Gamell LS, O'Donoghue MW, et al. Long-term changes in intraocular pressure after clear corneal phacoemulsification: normal patients versus glaucoma suspect and glaucoma patients. J Cataract Refract Surg. 1999;25:885-90.

6. Tennen DG, Masket S. Short-and long-term effect of clear corneal incisions on intraocular pressure. J Cataract Refract Surg. 1996;22:568-70.

7. Wedrich A, Menapace R, Radax U, Papapanos P. Long-term results of combined trabeculectomy and small incision cataract surgery. J Cataract Refract Surg. 1995;21:49-54.

8. Gimbel HV, Meyer D, DeBroff BM, et al. Intraocular pressure response to combined phacoemulsification and trabeculotomy ab externo versus phacoemulsification alone in primary open-angle glaucoma. J Cataract Refract Surg. 1995;21:653-60.

9. Agency for Healthcare Research and Quality. Evidence Report/ Technology Assessment. Number 38. Treatment of coexisting cataract and glaucoma. Washington, DC: AHRQ Publication No. 01-E049;2001.

10. Wyse T, Meyer M, Ruderman JM, et al. Combined trabeculectomy and phacoemulsification: a one-site vs a two-site approach. Am J Ophthalmol. 1998;125:334-9.

11. Park HJ, Weitzman M, Caprioli J. Temporal corneal phacoemulsification combined with superior trabeculectomy. A retrospective case-control study. Arch Ophthalmol. 1997;115:318-23.

12. Guillermo L, Urcelay-Segura JL, Ortega-Usobiaga J, et al. Combined catract extraction and filtering surgery. In: Agarawal S, Agarwal A, Agarwal A. Phacoemulsification, 3rd edition. 2004;2:596-608.

13. Lucio Burrato, Maurizio Zanini. Phacoemulsification in glaucomatous eyes. In: Lucio Buratto, Robert H Osher, Samuel Masket (eds). Cataract Surgery in Complicated Cases. Slack Inc. 2000.

14. Neuhann T, Ernest PH. Combined Phacoemulsification With Trabeculectomy. In: Lucio Buratto, Robert H Osher, Samuel Masket (eds). Cataract Surgery in Complicated Cases. Slack Inc. 2000.

15. Steve Obstbaum, Maurizio Zanini. Combined cataract and glaucoma surgery. In: Lucio Buratto, Robert H Osher, Samuel Masket (eds). Cataract Surgery in Complicated Cases. Slack Inc. 2000.

16. Sunita Agarwal, Sundaram, Asha B. Laser sclerotomy, laser phakonit and IOL implantation. In: Agarwal S, Agarwal A, Agarwal A. Phacoemulsification, 3rd edition. 2004. pp. 596-608.

17. Shin DH, Simone PA, Song MS, et al. Adjunctive subconjunctival mitomycin C in glaucoma triple procedure. Ophthalmology. 1995;102:1550-8.

18. Wong PC, Ruderman JM, Krupin T, et al. 5-Fluorouracil after primary combined filtration surgery. Am J Ophthalmol. 1994;117:149-54.

19. Higginbotham EJ, Stevens RK, Musch DC, et al. Bleb-related endophthalmitis after trabeculectomy with mitomycin C. Ophthalmology. 1996;103:650-6.
20. Greenfield DS, Suñer IJ, Miller MP, et al. Endophthalmitis after filtering surgery with mitomycin. Arch Ophthalmol. 1996;114:943-9.
21. Zacharia PT, Deppermann SR, Schuman JS. Ocular hypotony after trabeculectomy with mitomycin C. Am J Ophthalmol. 1993;16:314-26.
22. Costa VP, Wilson RP, Moster MR, et al. Hypotony maculopathy following the use of topical mitomycin C in glaucoma filtration surgery. Ophthalmic Surg. 1993;24:389-94.
23. Greenfield DS, Liebmann JM, Jee J, Ritch R. Late-onset bleb leaks after glaucoma filtering surgery. Arch Ophthalmol. 1998;116:443-7.
24. Friedrich Y, Raniel Y, Lubovsky E, Friedman Z. Late pigmented-membrane formation on silicone intraocular lenses after phacoemulsification with or without trabeculectomy. J Cataract Refract Surg. 1999;25:1220-5.
25. Jampel HD, Lubomski LH, Friedman DS, et al. Treatment of Coexisting Cataract and Glaucoma. Baltimore: Evidence-Based Practice Center, Johns Hopkins University, 6 Oct 2000. Contract No. 290-097-0006, Task Order 3.

The Malpositioned Intraocular Implant

Amar Agarwal, Clement K Chan, Priya Narang, Ashvin Agarwal

INTRODUCTION

Numerous advances in microsurgical techniques have led to highly safe and effective cataract surgery. Two of the current trends in the evolution of modern cataract techniques include increasingly smaller surgical incisions associated with phacoemulsification (e.g. sub 1.4 mm incisions as in phakonit with rollable IOL implantation),[1] as well as the movement from retrobulbar and peribulbar anesthesia to topical anesthesia, and even "no anesthesia" techniques.[2] Despite such advances, the malpositioning or dislocation of an intraocular lens (IOL) due to capsular rupture or zonnular dehiscence remains an infrequent but important sight-threatening complication for contemporary cataract surgery. The key to the prevention of poor visual outcome for this complication is its proper management. Many highly effective surgical methods have been developed to manage a dislocated IOL. They include manipulating the IOL with perfluorocarbon liquids, scleral loop fixation, using a snare, employing 25-gauge IOL forceps, temporary haptic externalization, as well as managing the one-piece plate IOL and two simultaneous intraocular implants.[3-13]

MANAGEMENT OF A MALPOSITIONED IOL

Disturbing visual symptoms such as diplopia, metamorphopsia, and hazy images are associated with a dislocated intraocular lens (IOL) (Fig. 8.1). If not properly managed, a malpositioned IOL may also induce sight-threatening ocular complications, including persistent cystoid macular edema, intraocular hemorrhage, retinal breaks, and retinal detachment. Contemporaneous with advances in phakonit microsurgical techniques for treating cataracts, a number of highly effective surgical methods have been developed for managing a dislocated IOL.

Chandelier Illumination

Visualization is done using a Chandelier illumination in which xenon light is attached to the infusion cannula. This gives excellent illumination and one can perform a proper bimanual vitrectomy as

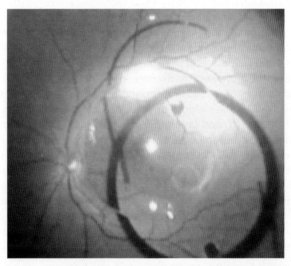

Figure 8.1 Dislocated IOL on the retina

an endoilluminator is not necessary for the surgeon to hold in the hand (Fig. 8.2). An inverter has to be used if one is using a wide field lens. The supermacula lens (Fig. 8.3) helps give better stereopsis so that one will not have any difficulty in holding the IOL with a diamond tipped forceps (Fig. 8.4). When one is using the Chandelier illumination system one hand can hold the IOL with the forceps and the other hand can hold a vitrectomy probe to cut the adhesions of the vitreous thus doing a bimanual vitrectomy (Fig. 8.5). One can also use two forceps to hold the lens thus performing a hand shake technique (Fig. 8.6). The lens is then brought out anteriorly and removed through the limbal route (Fig. 8.7).

Other techniques include IOL manipulation with perfluorocarbon liquids, scleral loop fixation, use of a snare, employing 25-Gauge IOL forceps, temporary haptic externalization, as well as managing the single plate implant and two simultaneous intraocular implants. The primary aim of such methods is to reposition the dislocated IOL close to the original site of the crystalline lens in an expeditious

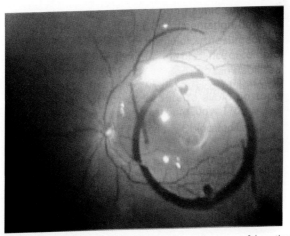

Figure 8.2 IOL lying over the macula. Notice the wide field view of the retina. This is because of the wide field contact lens being used and the Chandelier illumination which is seen in the upper left hand corner

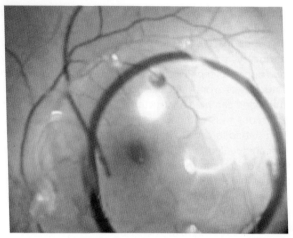

Figure 8.3 View using the super macula lens. This gives better stereopsis

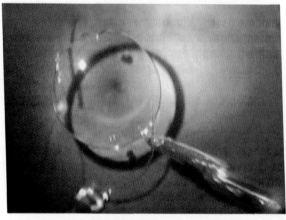

Figure 8.4 Diamond tipped forceps lifting a looped IOL lying on the retina after a vitrectomy

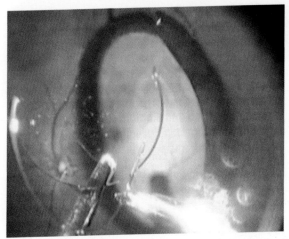

Figure 8.5 Forceps holding the IOL and the vitrectomy probe cutting the vitreous adhesions. This is bimanual vitrectomy which is possible due to the Chandelier illumination

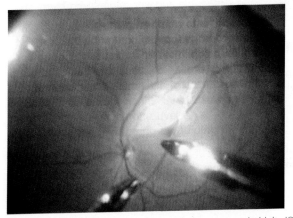

Figure 8.6 Handshake technique. Using two forceps one can hold the IOL comfortably and bring it anteriorly

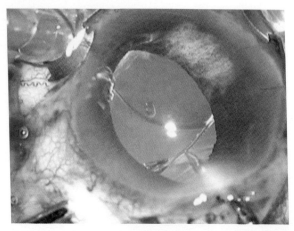

Figure 8.7 IOL brought out anteriorly through the limbal route. Notice in the upper right and left corners infusion cannulas fixed. One is for infusion and the other for the Chandelier illumination. One can also have the same infusion cannula with the Chandelier illumination

manner whenever possible, and with minimal morbidity, enhancing the chance of good visual outcome.

Perfluorocarbon Liquids

Chang popularized the use of perfluorocarbon liquids for the surgical treatment of various vitreoretinal disorders.[3] Due to their heavier-than-water properties, and their ease of intraocular injection and removal,[14-17] perfluorocarbon liquids are highly effective for flattening detached retina, tamponading retinal tears, limiting intraocular hemorrhage, as well as floating dropped crystalline lens fragments and a dislocated IOL.[18-25]

Types of Perfluorocarbon Liquids

Four types of perfluorocarbon liquids are frequently employed for intraocular surgery. They include:

1. Perfluoro-N-octane
2. Perfluoro-tributylamine
3. Perfluoro-decaline
4. Perfluoro-phenanthrene.
   Their physical properties are outlined in Table 8.1.

IOL Manipulation with Perfluorocarbon Liquids

Due to their unique physical properties, perfluorocarbon liquids are well suited for floating dropped lens fragments and dislocated IOL, in order to insulate the underlying retina from damages. At the same time, the anterior displacement of the dislocated IOL by the perfluorocarbon liquids facilitates its removal or repositioning.[18-27]

ACIOL

Dislocation of the ACIOL into the vitreous cavity is relatively infrequent in comparison to the PCIOL. However, the ACIOL may dislocate during trauma, particularly in the presence of a large sector iridectomy. A subluxated or posteriorly dislocated ACIOL

TABLE 8.1 Properties of perfluorocarbon liquids

Characteristic	Perfluoro-N-octane	Perfluoro-tributylamine	Perfluoro-decaline	Perfluoro-phenanthrene
Chemical formula	C3F18	C12F27N	C10F18	C14F24
Molecular weight	438	671	462	624
Specific gravity	1.76	1.89	1.94	2.03
Refractive index	1.27	1.29	1.31	1.33
Surface tension (Dyne/cm at 25°C)	14	16	16	16
Viscosity (Centistokes—25°C)	0.8	2.6	2.7	8.03
Vapor pressure (mm Hg at 37°C)	50	1.14	13.5	<1

may be simply repositioned into the anterior chamber.[28,29] If the dislocated ACIOL is attached to formed vitreous or is sitting deep in the posterior vitreous cavity, an initial partial vitrectomy to eliminate the vitreoretinal traction is preferred before the repositioning or removal of the ACIOL.[29] If there is any substantial anterior segment injury associated with the dislocation (e.g. marked iridodialysis, large hyphema, excessive angle damage, etc.), it is best to remove the dislocated ACIOL through a limbal incision.

Opened-Eye Or External Approach

This approach involves modifications of various suturing techniques for inserting an external primary or secondary PCIOL: sometimes in association with aphakic penetrating keratoplasty, or with an IOL exchange, in the absence of appropriate capsular or zonnular support.[30-50] The suture material can be easily tied to the externally located IOL before its re-insertion. A relatively large limbal incision is required for the externalization and the subsequent re-insertion of the entire dislocated PCIOL.

Closed-Eye Or Internal Approach—Pars Plana Techniques

This approach avoids the making of a large surgical incision that may induce undesirable astigmatism or tissue injury. The integrity of the globe is maintained, and the fluctuation of the intraocular pressure is minimized throughout the case. However, many internal techniques require the passage of sharp instruments or needles into the eye, which sometimes can be associated with the risk of an injury to the intraocular structures. Relatively intricate intraocular maneuvers may also be involved. In recent years, a number of internal techniques for the repositioning of the PCIOL with a pars plana approach have become increasingly popular.[4-11,25,26,51,52]

Scleral Loop Fixation

In 1991, Maguire and Blumenkranz, et al. described the preparation of a 9-0 or 10-0 polypropylene suture loop by making a simple knot or a series of twists on the suture with a pair of microforceps.[4] The same microforceps are used to grasp the suture adjacent to the suture loop for insertion through an anterior sclerotomy corresponding to the location of the ciliary sulcus, after a partial pars plana vitrectomy to eliminate the vitreoretinal traction. The inserted suture loop is then used to engage one of the dislocated haptics for anchoring at the anterior sclerotomy. The same maneuver is repeated for the opposite haptic.

The Grieshaber Snare

Grieshaber first manufactured a snare designed by Packo in the early 1990s. It consists of a 20-guage tube and a handle with a movable spring-loaded finger slide for adjusting the size of a protruding polypropylene loop. The distal portion of the tube with the polypropylene loop is inserted through an anterior sclerotomy for engaging a dislocated haptic in the vitreous cavity. Once the looped haptic is pulled up against the anterior sclerotomy, the external portion of the polypropylene loop is cut free and guided through a 30-guage needle for anchoring by the anterior sclerotomy. (Fig. 8.8). Little et al. reported the successful transscleral fixation of the dislocated PCIOL with the snare method in a series of cases in 1993.[5]

The 25-Gauge IOL Forceps

In 1994, Chang introduced the 25-gauge IOL forceps.[6] His passive-action forceps have smooth platforms at the distal end for grasping tissue or holding a suture, and a small groove at the proximal end for gripping a haptic.[6] After a partial vitrectomy, a sharp 25-gauge, 5/8 inch needle is inserted through a scleral groove at 0.8 mm posterior to the corneoscleral limbus, to create a tract for the 25-gauge forceps. The forceps holding a slipknot (lasso) on a 10-0 polypropylene suture is then inserted through the grooved scleral incision into the eye for engaging an IOL haptic. After looping the haptic, the forceps are released from the suture and are used to

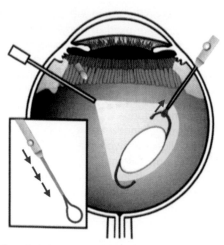

Figure 8.8 The grieshaber snare consists of a 20-guage tube and handle with a movable spring-loaded finger slide for adjusting the amount of a protruding polypropylene suture loop. The suture loop is inserted posteriorly to engage a dislocated haptic. The external portion of the suture loop is then cut free and guided through a 30-guage needle for anchoring at the sclera, after the engaged haptic is pulled up against the anterior sclerotomy

regrasp the end of the haptic; thus preventing the suture from slipping off the haptic. After tightening the slipknot, the IOL is repositioned in the ciliary sulcus by anchoring the needle of the 10-0 polypropylene suture within the scleral groove (Fig. 8.9). The same maneuver may be repeated for the opposite haptic, if necessary. The scleral groove is closed with an interrupted 10-0 nylon suture.

Temporary Haptic Externalization

Chan first described this method in 1992.[7] Its main features involve temporary haptic externalization for suture placement after a pars plana vitrectomy, followed by re-internalization of the haptics tied with 9-0 or 10-0 polypropylene sutures for secured anchoring by

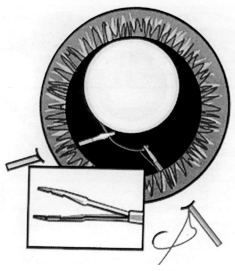

Figure 8.9 These 25-guage chang passive-action IOL forceps have smooth distal platforms for grasping tissues or sutures, and a proximal groove for gripping a haptic. A slip knot is inserted through a paralimbal scleral groove incision to engage the haptic of the IOL. The forceps are then used to regrasp the distal end of the haptic to prevent the slippage of the suture loop. After tightening the slip knot, the needle of the 10-0 polypropylene suture is anchored within the scleral groove for the implant fixation in the ciliary sulcus

the anterior sclerotomies.[7] The details of this technique include the following:[7,8]

- A 3-port pars plana vitrectomy is performed for the removal of the anterior and central vitreous adjacent to the dislocated IOL, in order to prevent any vitreoretinal traction during the process of manipulating the IOL.
- Two diametrically opposed limbal-based partial thickness triangular scleral flaps are prepared along the horizontal meridians at 3 and 9 o'clock. Anterior sclerotomies within the beds under the scleral flaps are made at 1 to 1.5 mm from the limbus (Fig. 8.10A). As an alternative to the scleral flaps, the

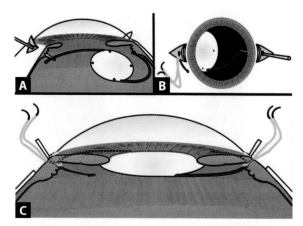

Figures 8.10A to C Temporary haptic externalization

anterior sclerotomies may be made within scleral grooves at 1 to 1.5 mm from the horizontal limbus.

- A fiberoptic light pipe is inserted through one of the posterior sclerotomies, while a pair of fine non-angled positive action forceps (e.g. Grieshaber) is inserted through the anterior sclerotomy of the opposing quadrant to engage one haptic of the dislocated IOL for temporary externalization (Fig. 8.10B). A double-armed 9-0 (Ethicon TG 160-8 plus, Somerville NJ) or 10-0 polypropylene suture (Ethicon CS 160-6 Somerville NJ) is tied around the externalized haptic to make a secured knot. The same process is repeated for the other haptic after the surgeon switches the instruments to his opposite hands.
- The externalized haptics with the tied sutures are re-internalized through the corresponding anterior sclerotomies with the same forceps (Fig. 8.10 C). The surgeon anchors the internalized haptics securely in the ciliary sulcus by taking scleral bites with the external suture needles on the lips of the anterior sclerotomies. By adjusting the tension of the opposing sutures while tying the polypropylene suture knots by the anterior sclerotomies, the

optic is centered behind the pupil, and the haptics are anchored in the ciliary sulcus.

Several important features of this technique include:[7,8]

- The horizontal meridians are chosen for the location of the anterior sclerotomies for easier manipulation of the forceps, haptics and sutures during the repositioning process.
- The locations of the anterior sclerotomies determine the final position of the IOL. Previous anatomic studies have reported the ciliary sulcus to be between 0.46 and 0.8 mm from the limbus.[53] Thus the distance of 1 to 1.5 mm from the limbus places the anterior sclerotomies close to the external surface of the ciliary sulcus. Making the anterior sclerotomies at less than 1 mm from the limbus increases the risk of injuring the anterior chamber angle or the iris root.
- The following steps are taken to ease the passage of the haptics through the anterior sclerotomies and reduce the chance of haptic breakage:
  - The anterior sclerotomies should have adequate size. If necessary, they may be widened before haptic reinternalization.
  - Fine nonangled positive action intraocular forceps are used for the haptic manipulation to give the surgeon the maximal "feel" and "control". Excessive pinching of the haptics is avoided during the passage of the haptics.

Several measures may also be taken to prevent the decentering and tilting of the IOL:

- The anterior sclerotomies are made at 180° from each other.
- The sutures are tied at equal distance from the ends of both haptics.
- A four-point fixation option: To enhance more stability, two separate polypropylene sutures can be tied on each haptic, and the associated needles are anchored on the two "corners" of each anterior sclerotomy. This allows a stable configuration of four-point fixation of the IOL.

This repositioning technique combines the best features of the external and the internal approaches, while avoiding any intricate and cumbersome intraocular manipulations. With the easy placement of the anchoring sutures in an "opened" environment and the maintenance of the integrity of the globe in a "closed" environment, this technique allows a precise and secured fixation of the dislocated IOL in the ciliary sulcus on a consistent basis.[7-9]

One Piece Silicone Plate IOL

There is a lack of fibrous adhesion between the lens capsule and the one-piece silicone IOL with plate haptics even years after its insertion into the capsular bag.[54-56] The "slippery" surface of the one-piece silicone plate implant makes it relatively mobile, even years after its placement. The silicone plate implant is fixated in the capsular bag by capsular contraction.[54-56] After its implantation, there is fibrotic fusion of the anterior and posterior capsules as well as capsular purse-stringing due to anterior capsular contraction.[54-56] These effects induce the posterior bowing of the silicone plate implant against the posterior capsule, resulting in the posterior capsular tightening and stretching.[54-56] Thus any dehiscence of the capsular bag outside of the capsulorhexis allows the release of the "built-up" tension, and the expulsion of the implant through the dehiscence.[10,11,54-56] Frequently, further capsular contraction after a posterior YAG capsulotomy may then vault the one-piece silicone plate implant through the opening into the vitreous cavity, in a delayed fashion.[10,11,54-56]

Previous reports have advocated the repositioning of the dislocated silicone plate implant anterior to the capsular remnants or in the ciliary sulcus.[10,11] Schneiderman and Johnson described the technique of picking the slippery silicone plate implant off the retinal surface with a lighted pick.[10,11] The surgeon extends the tip of the pick under the edge of the silicone plate implant to gently elevate it off the retinal surface. The elevated edge is then grasped with the intraocular forceps for the repositioning or removal of the implant. Alternatively, the plate implant may be brought anteriorly

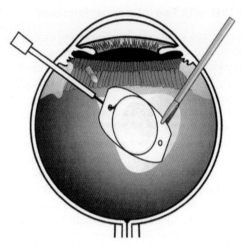

Figure 8.11 The slippery plate implant may be lifted on its edge or hooked through a positioning hole with a lighted pick, and then grasped with intraocular forceps for its repositioning or removal

by hooking the lighted pick through one of its positioning holes, and then grasped with forceps at the anterior or mid-vitreous cavity (Fig. 8.11). Another method is to aspirate the plate implant with a soft-tip cannula. As discussed above, perfluorocarbon liquids may also be used to float the dislocated plate implant. The one-piece silicone plate implant is designed for insertion into the capsular bag. Thus repositioning the silicone plate implant anterior to the capsular remnants or in the ciliary sulcus tends to be unstable, particularly without the support of sutures. None of the suturing methods (including the temporary haptic externalization technique described) work well for the one-piece silicone IOL with plate haptics. The temporary externalization of the bulky plate haptics of the silicone plate implant is awkward, and the suture placement through its "floppy" surface tends to result in the "cheese-wiring" of the implant. Frequently, the best approach for managing the dislocated one-piece silicone plate implant is its removal.

Managing Eyes with Two Intraocular Implants

The presence of two intraocular implants complicates the surgical management. This usually occurs when the cataract surgeon inserts a second implant (usually an ACIOL) without removing the posteriorly dislocated implant. If a dislocated implant is made out of relatively soft and inert material (e.g. one-piece silicone implant with plate haptics), it may not cause a retinal injury. In that situation, surgical intervention may be avoided, although intraocular movements of the loose implant may create a visual disturbance. Mobile dislocated implants with hard surfaces and sharp edges may induce an intraocular injury, and therefore should be removed. The association of vitreous hemorrhage, glaucoma, uveitis, retinal breaks, or a retinal detachment with the dislocated implant also requires surgical intervention. The presence of the second intraocular implant eliminates the option of repositioning the dislocated implant, and it also interferes with the removal of the dislocated implant. A number of techniques have been described in the removal of the dislocated implant in the presence of a second implant. The dislocated implant may be treated as an intraocular foreign body, and removed through a pars plana incision with standard vitreoretinal techniques, as reported by Williams et al.[12] The dislocated implant may also be removed through a limbal incision with or without the simultaneous removal of the second implant.[13] Wong recently described a technique of temporarily suspending the dislocated implant at the anterior vitreous cavity by passing a 6-0 nylon suture through one of the IOL positioning holes; followed by gently tilting up the edge of the second implant to allow the delivery of the dislocated implant out of the eye through a limbal incision.[13] Another option is the removal of the second implant followed by the repositioning of the dislocated implant. This option may be chosen if there is marked anterior segment pathology associated with a second anterior chamber implant (marked iridodialysis or hyphema, progressive corneal edema, etc.), and the dislocated posterior chamber implant can be safely fixated in the ciliary sulcus. The final option is the removal of both implants, particularly when the presence of any implant may aggravate a serious ocular condition; such as poorly controlled glaucoma, or an advanced retinal detachment with severe proliferative vitreoretinopathy. Whether the removal of one or both implants is through a limbal or pars plana opening, a relatively large incision is required, and complex maneuvers are necessary. This increases the chance of ocular morbidities. Thus the placement of a second implant should be avoided in the setting of a posteriorly dislocated implant.

SLEEVELESS EXTRUSION CANNULA ASSISTED LEVITATION OF DROPPED IOL

This technique[57] was started by Dr Ashvin Agarwal where in the sleeve of the extrusion cannula is removed before managing the dropped IOL. Removal of the silicon sleeve exposes wider access of the bore of the cannula, which helps to create an effective suction around the IOL.

After adequate vitrectomy is done (Fig. 8.12A), the sleeveless-extrusion cannula is connected to the vitreotome and the vacuum is set to 300 mm Hg, with the cutting function turned off. As the IOL rests flat on the retina, the sleeveless extrusion cannula is made to face the center of the optic and suction is initiated. The suction can be dynamically controlled with the foot pedal. The linear control of the foot pedal helps to increase the vacuum as and when needed during the levitation of IOL (Fig. 8.12B). Ineffective apposition of the lumen of the cannula to the surface of the IOL optic can lead to loss of vacuum. The IOL is lifted from the surface of the retina and is brought into the anterior vitreous in the mid-pupillary area (Fig. 8.12C). The end-opening forceps introduced from the corneal incision under direct visualization through the microscope grasps the IOL; the extrusion cannula is then removed as the forceps grasps the IOL. The IOL can then be subsequently managed depending on the surgical scenario. It can be either replaced or re-positioned in the sulcus or it can be explanted (Fig. 8.12D).

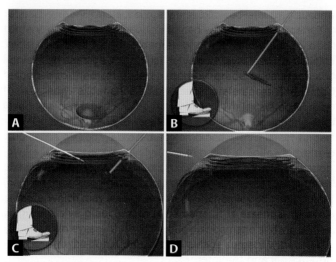

Figures 8.12A to D Technique of sleeveless extrusion cannula assisted levitation of dropped IOL: A. The IOL is lying flat on the retina; B. Sleeveless extrusion cannula is introduced into the eye and the bore of the cannula is made to face the surface of IOL. Suction is then generated with foot pedal in position 2 and the IOL is lifted; C. The IOL is brought into the mid-pupillary plane from where it is grasped by an end-opening forceps. The IOL is then brought into the anterior chamber and is then explanted; D. The IOL is explanted or repositioned depending on the presence or absence of sulcus support and also upon the type of IOL

The advantage with this technique is that it is safe, reliable and reproducible. Moreover, it is effective for dislocation of any type of IOL including the plate haptic IOLs which are often difficult to grasp with a retinal forceps.

SUMMARY

Capsular rupture or zonnular dehiscence during cataract surgery predisposes subsequent malpositioning or dislocation of an IOL. If the surgeon decides to insert a PC IOL after the loss of capsular or zonnular integrity, he should consider a large-diameter (6.0 or

6.5 mm) IOL, in order to decrease the chance of IOL malpositioning or dislocation. Placing the PC IOL in the ciliary sulcus or inserting an AC IOL may also diminish subsequent complications. The management of a malpositioned or dislocated intraocular implant is best accomplished via modern pars plana technology. The basic principles of management include initial anterior and posterior vitrectomy to eliminate any vitreous traction, followed by the use of various intraocular microforceps and small sutures to engage the dislocated IOL for its removal or repositioning. Due to their heavier-than-water properties, perfluorocarbon liquids are particularly valuable supplementary agents for manipulating the dislocated IOL in conjunction with various methods of IOL management. A dislocated AC IOL may be removed or repositioned. The repositioning of a dislocated PCIOL in the ciliary sulcus with modern vitreoretinal techniques provides the optimal environment for visual recovery. The PC IOL repositioning techniques may be broadly divided into the external and the internal approaches. The former involves modifications of suturing techniques for a primary or secondary implant in the absence of appropriate capsular or zonnular support, while the latter is best accomplished with pars plana technology. Some of the recent vitreoretinal methods of PCIOL repositioning gaining wide acceptance include scleral loop fixation,[24] the snare approach,[27] the use of perfluorocarbon,[30,32,33] employing the 25-guage implant forceps,[35] and temporary haptic externalization.[36] The temporary haptic externalization method combines the best features of the external and the internal approaches, avoids difficult intraocular maneuvers, and allows consistent IOL fixation in the ciliary sulcus. Unique features are associated with one-piece silicone plate implants. The capsular contraction after a posterior YAG capsulotomy often leads to a delayed posterior dislocation of the plate implant. Special techniques can be used to pick up the slippery plate implant from the retinal surface for its removal or repositioning. The plate implant repositioned anterior to capsular remnants or in the ciliary sulcus may be unstable, and it is often best to remove the dislocated plate implant. The placement of a second implant in the presence of a dislocated implant is ill advised, as it complicates subsequent surgical management. Surgical options include the removal of the dislocated implant through a pars plana or a limbal incision with special techniques, the repositioning of the dislocated implant after removing the second implant, or the removal of both implants. Surgical maneuvers in the setting of double implants are associated with increased morbidities and complications.

Key Points

- Disturbing visual symptoms such as diplopia, metamorphopsia, and hazy images are associated with a dislocated intraocular lens (IOL). If not properly managed, a malpositioned IOL may also induce sight-threatening ocular complications, including persistent cystoid macular edema, intraocular hemorrhage, retinal breaks, and retinal detachment.
- Due to their unique physical properties, perfluorocarbon liquids are well suited for floating dropped lens fragments and dislocated IOL, in order to insulate the underlying retina from damages.
- One excellent method is the use of a diamond tipped forceps to hold the IOL and bring it anteriorly after vitrectomy.
- The best method for visualization during vitrectomy is to use the Chandelier illumination system and use a wide field contact lens.
- Temporary haptic externalization involves temporary haptic externalization for suture placement after a pars plana vitrectomy, followed by re-internalization of the haptics tied with 9-0 or 10-0 polypropylene sutures for secured anchoring by the anterior sclerotomies.
- None of the suturing methods (including the temporary haptic externalization technique) work well for the one-piece silicone IOL with plate haptics.

REFERENCES

1. Agarwal A, Agarwal S, Agarwal A. Phakonit: Lens removal through a 0.9 mm incision. In: Agarwal A (ed). Phacoemulsification, Laser Cataract Surgery and Foldable IOL's, 1st edn. Jaypee Brothers Medical Publishers. 1998.

2. Agarwal A, Agarwal A, Agarwal S. No Anesthesia Cataract surgery. In: Agarwal A Phacoemulsification, Laser Cataract Surgery and Foldable IOL's Second edition. Jaypee Brothers Medical Publishers. 2000.

3. Chang S. Perfluorocarbon liquids in vitreo-retinal surgery. International Ophthalmology Clinics: New Approaches to Vitreoretinal Surgery. 1992;32(2):153-63.

4. Maguire AM, Blumenkranz MS, Ward TG, Winkelman JZ. Scleral loop fixation for posteriorly dislocated intraocular lenses. Operative technique and long-term results. Arch Ophthalmol. 1991;109:1754-8.

5. Little BC, Rosen PH, Orr G, Aylward GW. Trans-scleral fixation of dislocated posterior chamber intraocular lenses using a 9-0 microsurgical polypropylene snare. Eye. 1993;7:740-3.

6. Chang S, Coll GE. Surgical techniques for repositioning a dislocated intraocular lens, repair of iridodialysis, and secondary intraocular lens implantation using innovative 25-guage forceps. Am J Ophthalmol. 1995;119:165-74.

7. Chan CK, An improved technique for management of dislocated posterior chamber implants. Ophthalmol. 1992;99:51-7.

8. Chan CK, Agarwal A, Agarwal S, Agarwal A. Management of dislocated intraocular implants. In: Nagpal PN, Fine IH (eds). Ophthalmology Clinics of North America, Posterior Segment Complications of Cataract Surgery, December; Saunders WB Philadelphia. 2000.pp.681-93.

9. Thach AB, Dugel PU, Sipperley JO, Sneed SR, et al. Outcome of sulcus fixation of dislocated PCIOL's using temporary externalization of the haptics. [paper] AAO Annual Meeting, New Orleans, Louisiana, November 10. 1998.

10. Schneiderman TE, Johnson MW, Smiddy WE, Flynn HW Jr, et al. Surgical management of posteriorly dislocated silicone plate haptic intraocular lenses. Am J Ophthalmol. 1997;123:629-35.

11. Johnson MW, Schneiderman TE. Surgical management of posteriorly dislocated silicone plate intraocular lenses. Curr Opin Ophthalmol. 1998; 9:11-15.

12. Williams DF, Del Piero EJ, Ferrone PJ, Jaffe GJ, et al. Management of complications in eyes containing two intraocular lenses. Ophthalmol. 1998;105:2017-22.

13. Wong KL, Grabow HB. Simplified technique to remove posteriorly dislocated lens implants. Arch Ophthalmol. 2001;119:273-4.

14. Lakshminarayanan K, Venkataraman M. Physics. KCS Desikan and Co., Madras India. 1992.

15. Leopold LB, Davis KS. Life Science Library Water, Time Life International BV, USA. 1974.

16. Lapp RE. Life Science Library Matter, Time Life International BV, USA. 1974.

17. Subramanyam N, Lal B. A Textbook of BSc Physics. S Chand & Company Ltd, Delhi, India. 1985.

18. Glaser BM, Carter JB, Kuppermann BD, Michels RG. Perfluoro-octane in the treatment of giant retinal tears with proliferative vitreoretinopathy. Ophthalmology. 1991;98(11):1613-21.

19. Nabih M, Peyman GA, Clark Jr LC, Hoffman RE, Miceli M, AbouSteit M, et al. Experimental evaluation of perfluorophenanthrene as a high specific gravity vitreous substitute: A preliminary report. Ophthalmic Surgery. 1989;20:286-93.

20. Blinder KJ, Peyman GA, Paris CL, Dailey JP, Alturki W, LuiKwan-Rong, et al. Vitreon, a new perfluorocarbon. British Journal of Opthalmology. 1991;75:240-4.

21. Shapiro MJ, Resnick KI, Kim SH, Weinberg A. Management of the dislocated crystalline lens with a perfluorocarbon liquid. Am J Ophthalmol. 1991;112:401-5.

22. Liu K, Peyman GA, Chen M, Chang K. Use of high density vitreous substitute in the removal of posteriorly dislocated lenses or intraocular lenses. Ophthalmic Surg. 1991;22:503-7.

23. Lewis H, Blumenkranz MS, Chang S. Treatment of dislocated crystalline lens and retinal detachment with perfluorocarbon liquids. Retina. 1992; 12:299-304.

24. Rowson NJ, Bacon AS, Rosen PH. Perfluorocarbon heavy liquids in the management of posterior dislocation of the lens nucleus during phakoemulsification. Br J Ophthalmol. 1992;176(3):169-70.

25. Greve MD, Peyman GA, Mehta NJ, Millsap CM. Use of perfluoroperhydrophenanthrene in the management of posteriorly dislocated crystalline and intraocular lenses. Ophthalmic Surg. 1993; 24(9): 593-7.

26. Lewis H, Sanchez G. The use of perfluorocarbon liquids in the repositioning of posteriorly dislocated intraocular lenses. Ophthalmol. 1993;100:1055-9.

27. Elizalde J. Combined use of perfluorocarbon liquids and viscoelastics for safer surgical approach to posterior lens luxation [poster]. The Vitreous Society, 17th Annual Meeting, Sept, Rome Italy. 1999.pp.21-5.

28. Flynn HW Jr. Pars plana vitrectomy in the management of subluxated and posteriorly dislocated intraocular lenses. Graefes Arch Clin Exp Ophthalmol.1987;225:169-72.

29. Flynn HW Jr, Buus D, Culbertson WW. Management of subluxated and posteriorly dislocated intraocular lenses using pars plana vitrectomy instrumentation. J Cataract Refract Surg. 1990;16:51-6.

30. Jacobi KW, Krey H. Surgical management of intraocular lens dislocation into the vitreous: case report. J Am Intraocul Implant Soc. 1983; 9:58-9.

31. Mittra RA, Connor TB, Han DP, Koenig SB, et al. Removal of dislocated intraocular lenses using pars plana vitrectomy with placement of an open-loop, flexible anterior chamber lens. Ophthalmol. 1998;105:1011-4.

32. McCannel MA. A retrievable suture idea for anterior uveal problems. Ophthalmic Surg. 1976;7(2):98-103.

33. Stark WJ, Bruner WE. Management of posteriorly dislocated intraocular lenses. Ophthalmic Surg. 1980;11:495-7.

34. Sternberg P Jr, Michels RG. Treatment of dislocated posterior chamber intraocular lenses. Arch Ophthalmol. 1986;104:1391-3.

35. Girard L J. Pars plana phacoprosthesis (aphakic intraocular implant): a preliminary report. Ophthalmic Surg. 1981;12:19-22.

36. Girard L J, Nino N, Wesson M, et al. Scleral fixation of a subluxated posterior chamber intraocular lens. J Cataract Refract Surg. 1988;14:326-7.

37. Smiddy WE. Dislocated posterior chamber intraocular lens. A new technique of management. Arch Ophthalmol. 1989;107:1678-80.

38. Campo RV, Chung KD, Oyakawa RT. Pars plana vitrectomy in the management of dislocated posterior chamber lenses. Am J Ophthalmol. 1989;108:529-34.

39. Anand R, Bowman RW. Simplified technique for suturing dislocated posterior chamber intraocular lens to the ciliary sulcus [letter]. Arch Ophthalmol. 1990;108:1205-6.

40. Stark WJ, Goodman G, Goodman D, Gottsch J. Posterior chamber intraocular lens implantation in the absence of posterior capsular support. Ophthalmic Surg. 1988;19:240-3.

41. Hu BV, Shin DH, Gibbs KA, Hong YJ. Implantation of posterior chamber lens in the absence of posterior capsular and zonnular support. Arch Ophthalmol. 1988;106:416-20.

42. Shin DH, Hu BV, Hong YJ, Gibbs KA. Posterior chamber lens implantation in the absence of posterior capsular support [letter]. Ophthalmic Surg. 1988;19:606-7.

43. Dahan E. Implantation in the posterior chamber without capsular support. J Cataract Refract Surg. 1989;15:339-42.

44. Pannu JS. A new suturing technique for ciliary sulcus fixation in the absence of posterior capsule. Ophthalmic Surg. 1988;19:751-4.

45. Spigelman AV, Lindstrom RL, Nichols BD, et al. Implantation of a posterior chamber lens without capsular support during penetrating keratoplasty or as a secondary lens implant. Ophthalmic Surg. 1988;19:396-8.

46. Drews RC. Posterior chamber lens implantation during keratoplasty without posterior lens capsule support. Cornea. 1987;6:38-40.

47. Wong SK, Stark WJ, Gottsch SD, et al. Use of posterior chamber lenses in pseudophakic bullous keratopathy. Arch Ophthalmol. 1987;105:856-8.

48. Waring GO III, Stulting RD, Street D. Penetrating keratoplasty for pseudophakic corneal edema with exchange of intraocular lenses. Arch Ophthalmol. 1987;105:58-62.

49. Shin DH. Implantation of a posterior chamber lens without capsular support during penetrating keratoplasty or as a secondary lens [letter]. Ophthalmic Surg. 1988;19:755-6

50. Lindstrom RL, Harris WS, Lyle WA. Secondary and exchange posterior chamber lens implantation. J Am Intraocul Implant Soc. 1982; 8:353-6.

51. Bloom SM, Wyszynski RE, Brucker AJ. Scleral fixation suture for dislocated posterior chamber intraocular lens. Ophthalmic Surg. 1990; 21:851-4.

52. Friedberg MA, Pilkerton AR. A new technique for repositioning and fixating a dislocated intraocular lens. Arch Ophthalmol. 1992;110:413-5.

53. Duffey RJ, Holland EJ, Agapitos PJ, Lindstrom RL. Anatomic study of transsclerally sutured intraocular lens implantation. Am J Ophthalmol. 1989;108:300-9.

54. Milauskas AT. Posterior capsule opacification after silicone lens implantation and its management. J Cataract Refract Surg. 1987;13:644-8.

55. Milauskas AT. Capsular bag fixation of one-piece silicone lenses. J Cataract Refract Surg. 1990;16:583-6.

56. Joo CK, Shin JA, Kim JH. Capsular opening contraction after continuous curvilinear capsulorhexis and intraocular lens implantation. J Cataract Refract Surg. 1996;22:585-90.

57. Agarwal A, Narang P, Agarwal A, Kumar DA. Sleeveless-extrusion cannula for levitation of dislocated intraocular lens. Br J Ophthalmol. 2014;98(7):910-4.

Managing Dislocated Lens Fragments

Clement K Chan, Amar Agarwal, Priya Narang

INTRODUCTION

Dislocation of lens fragments into the vitreous cavity occurs in a small percentage of cases of cataract extraction with phacoemulsification or phakonit but continues to be encountered on an intermittent basis with potentially serious consequences in the modern setting.[1] Small lens fragments consisting of mostly cortical material may gradually resolve with conservative medical management alone. However, large lens fragments with a sizeable nuclear component do not resolve easily, and may elicit a phacoantigenic response from the host.[2-5] The released lens proteins may not only induce persistent intraocular inflammation, but also block the trabecular meshwork, resulting in phacolytic (or lens particle) glaucoma.[6,7] In time, other serious anatomical complications with poor visual consequences may develop in the absence of appropriate management of the lens fragments, i.e. peripheral anterior synechiae of the iris, pupillary or vitreous membranes, cystoid macular edema, retinal breaks or detachment, and phacoanaphylaxis, etc.[1-5] Therefore, most retained and dislocated lens fragments with a substantial nuclear component require surgical removal.[1,5,8-10] Earlier clinical studies advocated the immediate removal of dislocated lens fragments.[11,12] In Blodi's report, those eyes undergoing surgery within 7 days had a lower incidence of long-term glaucoma.[11] However, subsequent reports by Gilliland et al. and Kim et al. demonstrated no difference in visual outcome and glaucoma development between those eyes undergoing lens fragment removal within 7 days and those after 30 days following the dislocation.[13,14] Despite such conclusions, expeditious surgical management of retained lens fragments within a limited time frame is the current standard of care that allows rapid visual rehabilitation and prevention of serious complications mentioned above.[1,11,12,14]

THE RESPONSIBILITY OF THE CATARACT SURGEON

In the event of a rupture of the posterior lens capsule or zonular dehiscence leading to posterior migration of lens fragments, the cataract surgeon must avoid any uncontrolled and forceful surgical maneuvers in the vitreous cavity in an attempt to retrieve the sinking lens fragments. Any retrieval technique that does not provide for the appropriate management of the vitreous first creates the potential of immediate or subsequent retinal complications. Thus, the cataract surgeon must refrain from the temptation of passing a sharp instrument or lens loop into the mid or posterior vitreous cavity to engage the sinking lens fragments, or passing forceful irrigation fluid into the vitreous cavity to float the lens fragments.[1,15,16] Such maneuvers usually generate vitreoretinal traction resulting in retinal breaks and detachment. Instead, he should finish the clean up of the remaining cortical debris within the capsular bag and its vicinity, and then also perform a limited anterior vitrectomy in the event of vitreous prolapse into the anterior chamber and at the cataract wound.[1,5,11-14,16,17] An intraocular lens (IOL) may also be implanted in the absence of significant anterior segment complications, i.e. corneal decompensation, iridodialysis, hyphema, anterior chamber angle injury, etc.[1,13,14,16,17] An anterior chamber intraocular lens (ACIOL) can usually be safely implanted, but it may induce postoperative corneal pathology, chronic cystoid macular edema, and even glaucoma under certain circumstances.[18] Frequently, a posterior chamber IOL (PCIOL) implant can be safely inserted at the ciliary sulcus or even into the capsular bag with the aid of a capsular tension ring for cases with limited capsular or zonular damages.[18-20] The surgeon should avoid the implantation of an IOL made of silicone material due to its potential of interfering with subsequent vitreoretinal surgery, particularly in the event of fluid-gas exchange or long term silicone oil tamponade.[21] The moisture condensation on the posterior surface of a silicone IOL due to its hydrophobic properties leads to a loss of visibility during fluid-gas exchange,[21] and silicone oil may erode into the silicone IOL with long term silicone oil tamponade subsequently. In addition, the surgeon should avoid the implantation of an IOL altogether in the presence of a rock-hard dislocated lens fragment, which may need to be removed intact through a limbal incision subsequently (see sections on cryoextraction and perfluorocarbon liquid).[1,17] Finally, a watertight wound closure is important in anticipation of postoperative intraocular pressure fluctuation and subsequent posterior surgical maneuvers for the lens fragments.[1,17] With the completion of the anterior segment maneuvers described above, the cataract surgeon is now ready to consider various options for managing the posteriorly dislocated lens fragments. In case of familiarity with vitreoretinal techniques, he may convert over to a posterior segment set-up and utilize one of the methods described in the following sections for removing the lens fragments. Otherwise, a prompt referral of the patient to a vitreoretinal surgeon is recommended. At the same time, medical management with topical anti-inflammatory, antibiotic, as well as cycloplegic medications should be instituted. If necessary, hypotensive agents are also utilized.

TECHNIQUES FOR REMOVING POSTERIORLY DISLOCATED LENS FRAGMENTS

Sleeveless Phacotip Assisted Levitation (SPAL)

This innovative method was introduced by Agarwal et al. and was previously known as FAVIT.[22] Its major advantage is that it allows the cataract surgeon familiar with vitreoretinal techniques to quickly convert over to posterior segment surgery with a limited amount of additional setup of instrumentation for removing the lens fragments. FAVIT stands for (FA—fallen and VIT—vitreous) meaning a technique to remove fragments fallen into the vitreous. A better term was then coined for this method and it came to be known as SPAL. Standard 3-port pars plana vitrectomy incisions are framed (Fig. 9.1) and an infusion cannula is fixated through the first port. An endoilluminator is then inserted through the second port, and a vitrectomy probe is inserted through the third port. Next, the surgeon performs a thorough posterior vitrectomy including the elimination of the vitreous fibers surrounding the retained lens fragments, in order to prevent subsequent vitreoretinal traction. After the completion of the posterior vitrectomy, the surgeon replaces the vitrectomy probe with a phacoemulsification probe (sleeveless) through the same incision. With the ultrasonic power at 50% and the aspiration intensity at moderate setting, the surgeon activates the suction-only mode to elevate the lens fragment from the retinal surface.

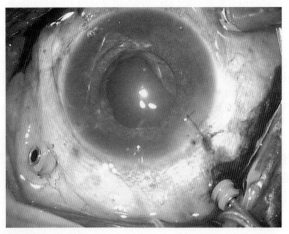

Figure 9.1 Standard 3-port pars plana vitrectomy incisions are framed

He quickly applies a small burst of ultrasonic energy to embed the probe tip into the elevated lens fragment (Fig. 9.2), and then lifts the entire fragment anteriorly. The endoilluminator is also used at the same time to guide the lens fragment above the iris plane and into the anterior chamber (Fig. 9.3). Once the lens fragment is in the anterior chamber, an IOL scaffold procedure can be performed where a 3-piece IOL is implanted below the lens fragments and is dialed over the residual capsular support (Figs 9.4 and 9.5). In cases of inadequate sulcus support, the IOL can even be placed above the iris and the nucleus can be emulsified. The optic of the IOL acts as scaffold and prevents any loss of lens fragments into the posterior cavity. The same IOL can then be fixed in the eye by glued IOL procedure. Stromal hydration is done to secure the corneal wound and air bubble is injected into the anterior chamber (Fig. 9.6).

In cases of hard cataract, the corneal section can be enlarged and the nucleus can then be expelled from the eye as in a routine extracapsular cataract surgery.

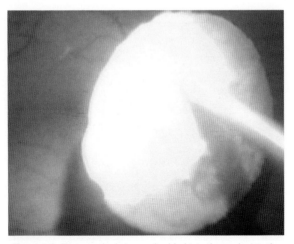

Figure 9.2 Phaco probe being embedded into the nucleus in the mid-vitreous cavity

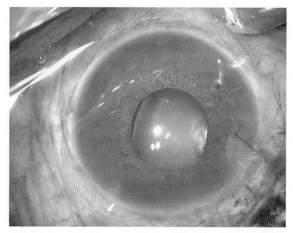

Figure 9.3 The nucleus is levitated and brought into the mid-pupillary plane

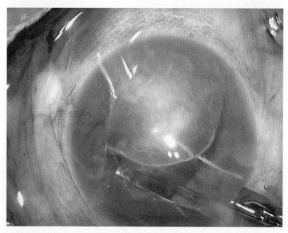

Figure 9.4 Nucleus in anterior chamber. A 3-piece foldable IOL being injected beneath the nucleus

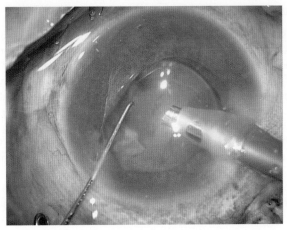

Figure 9.5 The nucleus being emulsified with a phaco probe

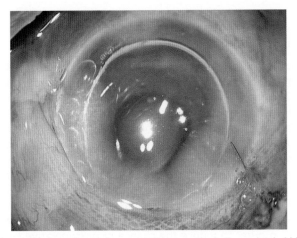

Figure 9.6 Corneal wounds secured with stromal hydration and air bubble injected in the anterior chamber

Vitrectomy and Phacofragmentation Techniques

The standard three-port pars plana vitrectomy approach is the most frequently employed method for the removal of posteriorly dislocated lens fragments in a safe and effective manner.[1,5,8-14,16,17] The first step involves the insertion of a posterior infusion cannula at the inferior temporal pars plana. In the event of a localized concomitant choroidal detachment in the inferior temporal quadrant, an alternative quadrant (e.g. inferior nasal) may be chosen for the infusion cannula. Frequently, cloudy media resulting from dense lens fragments or in some cases hyphema and fibrin deposits surrounding the implant, may prevent an adequate view of the tip of the pars plana infusion cannula. In that situation, the surgeon may ascertain the proper intravitreal location of the infusion cannula tip by inserting a microvitreoretinal blade through one of the superior pars plana sclerotomies to rub against the cannula tip, before turning on the infusion fluid. Utilizing a longer infusion cannula (e.g. 4- or 6-mm) is also advantageous in avoiding inadvertent subretinal or choroidal infusion.

Managing the Anterior Chamber Opacities and Herniated Vitreous

Cloudy lens material, hemorrhagic infiltrates, and fibrin deposits in the anterior chamber must be first eliminated before the performance of a posterior vitrectomy and phacofragmentation.[1,5,16,17] For the anterior chamber washout, a separate infusion cannula (e.g. a 20- or 22-gauge angled rigid or flexible soft cannula) may be inserted at the limbus for anterior chamber infusion and prevention of chamber collapse. Microsurgical picks, hooks, bent needle tips, or forceps may be used to remove opaque membranes from the anterior and posterior surfaces of the implant.[1] Vitreous herniated into the anterior chamber and vitreous strands attached to the iris or the limbal surgical wound must be excised with a vitrectomy probe in order to reduce the chance of postoperative cystoid macular edema and other types of vitreoretinal complications. To further enhance anterior media clarity, intracameral viscoelastic substances can be injected to coat the corneal endothelium for reducing striate keratopathy, displace blood from the visual axis, or to achieve hemostasis associated with a persistent hyphema.[1,5] Unwanted residual lenticular capsular remnants may also be eliminated with the vitrectomy probe. Pupillary dilation may be maintained throughout surgery with the administration of topical and subconjunctival mydriatics, or intracameral epinephrine.[1,5] If necessary, temporary iris retractors can be inserted via multiple limbal incisions to maintain pupillary dilation during surgery.

Posterior Vitrectomy and Phacofragmentation

After completing the core vitrectomy, it is important for the surgeon to carefully remove all of the vitreous fibers surrounding the posterior lens fragments before proceeding with phacofragmentation, in order to prevent the occlusion of the phaco tip by formed vitreous elements during the phacofragmentation process and also prevent traction on the retina.[1,5,8-14,16,17] In fact, the surgeon should remove as much of the vitreous as he can safely achieve before performing phacoemulsification, in order to avoid unwanted vitreoretinal traction.[16] Perfluorocarbon liquid may be infused into the eye to serve as a cushion for protecting the underlying retina from the bouncing lens fragments during the process of lens emulsification (Fig. 9.7). Only a limited amount of perfluorocarbon liquid should be injected, since excessive perfluorocarbon liquid with a convex meniscus tends to displace the lens fragments away from the central visual axis and toward the peripheral fundus and the vitreous base.[1] In case of peripheral displacement of the lens fragments, a layer of viscoelastic may be applied on top of the perfluorocarbon liquid to neutralize its convex meniscus, resulting in recentering of the lens fragments toward the visual axis, a simple maneuver described by Elizalde (Fig. 9.8).[23]

At the start of the pars plana phacoemulsification process, each lens fragment is first engaged at the phaco tip with the machine set at the aspiration mode and then brought to the mid vitreous

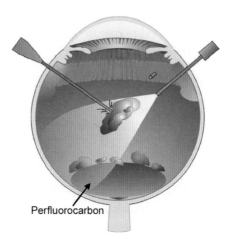

Perfluorocarbon

Figure 9.7 Insulating the retina with perfluorocarbon: A small amount of perfluorocarbon liquid may be infused on the retinal surface to protect it from dropped lens fragments during the process of lens emulsification. Excessive perfluorocarbon is avoided to decrease the propensity of peripheral displacement of the floating lens fragments toward the vitreous base due to the convex meniscus of the perfluorocarbon. During phacoemulsification, the ultrasonic power of the phaco probe is kept at a low to medium setting to reduce the tendency of blowing the lens fragments from the phaco tip toward the retina

cavity for emulsification.[16,17,24] During the emulsification of the lens fragments, the ultrasonic power is kept at a low or moderate setting in order to decrease the tendency of blowing the fragments from the phaco tip and repeatedly dropping them on the retina.[16,17] The more advanced phacofragmentation units with sophisticated linear (proportional) ultrasonic and aspiration controls tend to reduce the erratic movements of the lens fragments at the phaco tip during the fragmentation process. The surgeon may also stabilize a large lens fragment in the mid-vitreous cavity by using his other hand to spear the fragment with an endoilluminator with a hook or pick at its tip for emulsification (Fig. 9.9).[1,12] As an alternative, he may utilize the bimanual "crush" or "chopstick" technique, which involves the use of his other hand to methodically crush each lens fragment with the

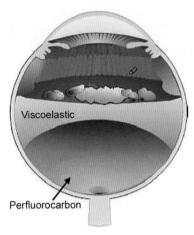

Figure 9.8 Recentering lens fragments on top of perfluorocarbon with viscoelastic: A layer of viscoelastic is applied on top of the perfluorocarbon liquid to neutralize its convex surface meniscus for recentering a peripherally displaced lens fragment toward the visual axis. (*Courtesy* of Elizalde J, 1999; modified and published with permission)

tip of an endoilluminator against the phaco tip before aspirating it from the eye through the phaco tip (Fig. 9.10).[1,16] After emulsifying and removing the bulk of the lens fragments, the surgeon eliminates any remaining vitreous with the vitrectomy probe. He also carefully searches for and removes residual small lens fragments embedded at the vitreous base, as well as inspects the peripheral fundus with indirect ophthalmoscopy.[1] One can use a combination of perfluorocarbon liquids and FAVIT also (Figs 9.11 to 9.14). In this once vitrectomy is done PFCL is injected to raise the nuclear fragments from the retinal level. Then using the phaco needle they are removed. Retinal breaks and peripheral retinal detachment discovered during the inspection are then promptly treated with the appropriate modality (e.g. laser, cryotherapy, scleral buckling, fluid-air or gas exchange, etc.) Residual perfluorocarbon liquid is removed before closure. The postoperative therapy includes the

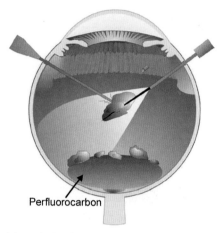

Perfluorocarbon

Figure 9.9 Stabilizing the lens fragment with a sharp instrument for emulsification: The surgeon may stabilize a lens fragment in the mid-vitreous cavity by using his other hand to spear the fragment with an endoilluminator probe with a hook or pick at its tip for emulsification

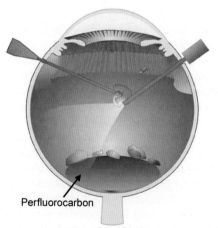

Perfluorocarbon

Figure 9.10 Crush method: The surgeon may also use his other hand to methodically crush each lens fragment with the endoilluminator tip against the phaco tip, before aspirating it from the eye through the phaco tip

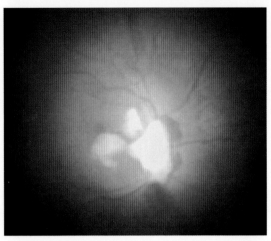

Figure 9.11 Combination of perfluorocarbon liquid (PFCL) and FAVIT (*Courtesy:* Dr Agarwal's Eye Hospital). Small nuclear fragments are lying on the retina

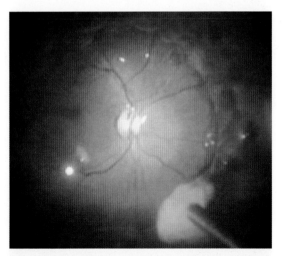

Figure 9.12 Combination of perfluorocarbon liquid (PFCL) and FAVIT (*Courtesy:* Dr Agarwal's Eye Hospital). Perfluorocarbon liquid is injected once vitrectomy is done. Then using the phaco needle the nuclear pieces are removed

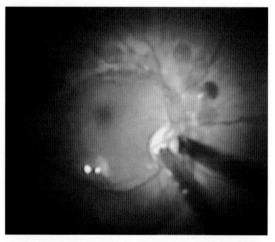

Figure 9.13 Combination of perfluorocarbon liquid (PFCL) and FAVIT (*Courtesy:* Dr Agarwal's Eye Hospital). The perfluorocarbon liquid is then aspirated

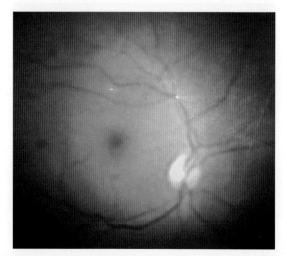

Figure 9.14 Combination of perfluorocarbon liquid (PFCL) and FAVIT (*Courtesy:* Dr Agarwal's Eye Hospital). The retina as seen once the case is completed

application of topical steroidal or nonsteroidal anti-inflammatory medications, antibiotics, and cycloplegics.

Previous studies utilizing the phacoemulsification methods similar to the above description reported favorable visual outcome (i.e. a final visual acuity of 20/40 or better with 52 to 87% of treated eyes).[12-14,25]

Endoscopic Technique

The endoscopic approach is best suited for removing dislocated lens fragments from eyes with an opacified cornea, a miotic or occluded pupil, persistent hyphema, or a cloudy IOL, etc.[26-33] It also provides a clear and unimpeded view of lens fragments trapped at the vitreous base. It allows the surgeon to scrutinize peripheral fundus details and appreciate the precise anatomical relationship of various retro-irideal structures (e.g. irido-capsular interface, haptic-ciliary junction, vitreous base, etc.) The magnified and undistorted images of the peripheral intraocular structures provided by the endoscope cannot be obtained through other methods. The endoscopic system includes an endoscopic hand piece with a probe, connected to a fiberoptic light source, a charged coupled device (CCD) video camera system and recorder, coupled with a high-resolution color video monitor.[26-33] For optimal viewing, a bright light source such as Xenon is preferred, although halogen lights can be used.[26-33] The two types of ophthalmic endoscopic systems that are commercially available include the gradient index (GRIN) solid-rod endoscopes first developed by Eguchi,[26,27] and the fiberoptic endoscopes subsequently developed by Uram and Fisher.[27-31] Both types of devices share the principle of image acquisition and optics transfer through the distal probe, and then image magnification and coupling in the handpiece or the remote CCD camera unit (Fig. 9.15A).[27] The GRIN solid rod endoscope employs a single long, slender, glass lens for optics transfer. The image acquired at the probe is transmitted along the length of a cylindrical pathway of the solid lens with a gradient index in a sinusoidal mode to a CCD camera unit (Fig. 9.15B).[26,27] The index of refraction of the lens varies with the

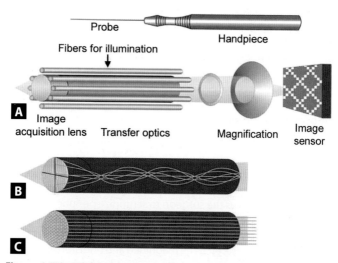

Figures 9.15A to C Principle of an ophthalmic endoscopic system: A. The image acquired at the tip of an endoscopic handpiece is transmitted through an optical pathway (GRIN solid-lens or a fiberoptic bundle). The image magnification and coupling to the CCD camera system take place at the proximal portion of the handpiece and the CCD camera unit; B. GRIN endoscope: The image acquired at the probe is transmitted along the length of a cylindrical pathway of the solid lens with a gradient index (index of refraction varies with the distance from the central axis) in a sinusoidal mode to a CCD camera unit; C. Fiberoptic endoscope: The image acquired with a GRIN lens at the distal end of a handpiece is transferred through a bundle of microfibers (via total internal reflection within each fiber) to a CCD camera unit

distance from the central axis. In the case of a fiberoptic endoscope, the image acquired with a GRIN lens at the distal end of a handpiece is transferred through a bundle of microfibers (via total internal reflection within each fiber) to a CCD camera unit (Fig. 9.15C).[27-32] The fiberoptic endoscope allows for a lighter handpiece. However, its image resolution is limited by the pixel density of the CCD camera as well as the density of the microfibers, and its depth of field is less than the GRIN single-rod endoscope.[27] Besides vitrectomy and phacoemulsification, other surgical maneuvers including laser photocoagulation can be performed in conjunction with the endoscopic system.[27-29] Laser componentry can be built into the endoscopic system.[27-29] For instance, the endoscopic hand piece may contain an optical path for viewing, besides separate fibers for endoillumination and photocoagulation. Thus a single endoscopic handpiece can be constructed with the capability of performing multiple tasks simultaneously: viewing, endoillumination, and photocoagulation.[27-29] Even a channel for infusion can also be incorporated into the endoscope.[27] However, the multiple functions increase the bulk and weight of the hand piece. One commercially available fiberoptic endoscopic system offers a 20-gauge endoscopic hand piece with a 3000-pixel fiberoptic bundle allowing a 70-degree field of view and a depth of focus from 0.5 to 7.0 mm, or an 18-gauge hand piece with a 10,000-pixel fiberoptic bundle allowing a 110-degree field of view and a depth of focus from 1 to 20 mm.[28,29] Drawbacks of the endoscopic method include the lack of a stereoscopic or three-dimensional view, and an initially steep learning curve for the surgeon.[1,33] Excellent surgical results can be achieved with this technique. In their study published in 1998, Boscher and associates reported consistently successful outcome in the use of the endoscopic method for managing a consecutive series of 30 eyes with dislocated lens fragments or IOLs.[33]

Further development in ophthalmic endoscopic systems holds the promise of providing unparalleled microscopic images of intraocular structures (even on a cellular level) that are not possible through conventional surgical instrumentation (e.g. viewing of sensory retinal, retinal pigment epithelial, and choroidal components in the subretinal space during vitreoretinal surgery.)[27] The construction of stereoscopic endoscopes is also technically feasible.

Removal by Cryoextraction

This method is reserved for removing an entire dislocated lens or a large and particularly hard lens nucleus that would otherwise require application of excessive intraocular ultrasonic energy and time-consuming manipulation with the conventional phacoemulsification approach.[24,34,35] When properly performed, it allows rapid delivery of a hard lens nucleus from the retinal surface to the anterior chamber and then out of the eye through a limbal incision, in the absence of an intraocular implant obstructing the passage of the lens nucleus. It is critical that the surgeon first performs a meticulous vitrectomy to eliminate all vitrolenticular and vitreoretinal traction. A fluid-air exchange is also required immediately before the insertion of the endocryoprobe to engage the dislocated lens nucleus.[1,24] The surgeon's failure to eliminate sufficient vitreous fluid from the eye before activation of the endocryoprobe may result in spreading of the freezing ice-ball throughout the residual vitreous fluid and the adjacent retina. Thus this seemingly simple surgical approach is associated with multiple potential hazardous complications. While delivering the hard lens nucleus anteriorly, the surgeon must apply a continuous freeze of sufficient intensity on the lens fragment to prevent its fall from the probe, but at the same time, avoid an excessive freeze that may damage the surrounding vital intraocular structures, including the retina, iris, and cornea, etc. This delicate balance and the intrinsically unpredictable behavior of the expanding ice-ball present a difficult challenge to the surgeon, particularly in the presence of poor visibility through a hazy cornea frequently encountered in such cases made even worse by the intraocular air.[1,35] Due to its potential of inducing retinal necrosis, vitreous hemorrhage, and even severe choroidal and expulsive hemorrhage, it is the authors' opinion that posterior cryoextraction should be limited to select cases of large dislocated hard lens nuclei and performed with extreme caution by an experienced surgeon.

Manipulation with Perfluorocarbon Liquid

High density, inert behavior, and low viscosity are unique properties of perfluorocarbon liquid that allow its use as an elegant surgical tool for removing dislocated lens fragments with minimal instrumentation in a safe and consistent manner.[35-38] As described in the previous section, perfluorocarbon liquid is frequently used to insulate the retina from injury by dropped lens fragments during phacoemulsification.[1] Perfluorocarbon is particularly effective when the surgeon is faced with the adverse condition of poor visibility through a hazy cornea and a dislocated nucleus with a rock-hard consistency.[1,35] In that situation, he may use perfluorocarbon alone without phacoemulsification to deliver the lens fragment anteriorly for its extraction through a limbal wound. Employing conventional phacoemulsification techniques to retrieve a hard lens nucleus may be time consuming and hazardous, particularly in the presence of marked ocular inflammation and a cloudy media with poor visibility.[35] Historically, several methods of removing a dislocated hard nucleus were utilized in the past.[35,39,40] With the exception of cryoextraction, these methods have been largely abandoned due to their technical difficulties and associated potential complications. They include trapping the lens nucleus with two needles passed across the globe with the patient in a prone position and buoying the lens nucleus anteriorly with sodium hyaluronate.[35,39,40] The needle-trapping technique is inherently difficult to apply and is associated with many potential hazards.[35,39] Although sodium hyaluronate is well tolerated by the eye, its relatively low density in comparison to perfluorocarbon does not allow the buoying of the lens nucleus on a consistent basis.[35] In contrast to perfluorocarbon liquid, clear visibility is required for the precise placement of the sodium hyaluronate with a cannula under the dislocated nucleus in order for it to float the nucleus. To avoid the premature dilution and extrusion of the sodium hyaluronate from the globe, the infusion fluid must also be turned off temporarily during the placement of the sodium hyaluronate. Such a maneuver may lead to hypotony and miosis with potentially serious consequences during surgery.[35,40] For the above reasons, perfluorocarbon liquid is superior to sodium hyaluronate and is currently the agent of choice for floating a posteriorly dislocated lens fragment for removal.[35-38]

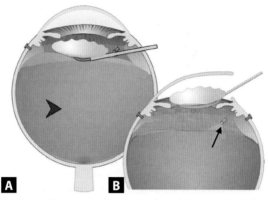

Figures 9.16A and B Removal of entire hard lens fragment with perfluorocarbon: A. After a thorough clean up of the anterior lenticular remnants and a posterior vitrectomy to eliminate vitreoretinal traction, perfluorocarbon liquid (arrowhead) is infused via a pars plana sclerotomy into the vitreous cavity to float the hard lens fragment, until it is lodged at the vitreous base between the surface of the perfluorocarbon and the iris as well as the ciliary processes. A soft-tipped cannula is inserted through a sclerotomy to recenter the lens fragment behind the pupil; B. Slow infusion of balanced salt solution (arrow) on top of the perfluorocarbon allows the gentle floating of the lens fragment further anteriorly. A lens loop is then used to carefully bring the lens fragment into the anterior chamber for delivery out of the eye through a limbal incision (modified and reprinted from Am J Ophthalmol, Volume 112, Shapiro et al. Management of the dislocated crystalline lens with a perfluorocarbon liquid, Pages 401-405, Figures 3 and 4, 1991, with permission from Elsevier Science)

Shapiro and associates reported the removal of dislocated hard lens nuclei with perfluoro-n-octane in 1991 (Figs 9.16A and B).[35] Their technique includes an initial vitrectomy to eliminate vitreoretinal traction after a thorough clean up of the anterior lenticular cortical and capsular remnants. The subsequent intraocular infusion of perfluoro-n-octane floats the hard lens nucleus anteriorly toward the vitreous base. The nuclear fragment is displaced peripherally due to the convex meniscus of the perfluorocarbon, and temporarily wedged at the vitreous base between the surface of the perfluorocarbon and the iris and ciliary processes. No attempt is made to directly expulse the dislocated lens fragment into the anterior chamber and out of the limbal wound with the perfluorocarbon liquid, due to potential mechanical injury of the corneal endothelium and the iris by the hard lens nucleus with such a maneuver. Instead, a soft-tipped cannula is inserted through a sclerotomy to recenter the lens nucleus behind the pupil (Fig. 9.16A). The lens nucleus is then gently floated further anteriorly with slow infusion of balanced salt solution on top of the perfluorocarbon, and carefully brought into the anterior chamber for delivery out of the eye with a lens loop through a limbal incision (Fig. 9.16B). In the absence of poor integrity of the cornea and the iris, a secondary IOL can be conveniently implanted through the same limbal incision before closure. Due to its low viscosity and tendency for posterior pooling, the surgeon can easily remove the perfluorocarbon liquid with a small aspiration cannula after the closure of the limbal wound at the end of surgery. Besides Shapiro's report, there have been a series of reports by multiple surgeons in the effective use of a variety of perfluorocarbon liquids to remove dislocated intraocular lens fragments. Similar to cryoextraction, this method of removing lens fragments is not appropriate for an eye with an IOL, unless the IOL is explanted first or at the time of the lens fragment removal.

The special properties of perfluorocarbon liquid make it especially suitable as an intraocular tool for atraumatic tissue manipulation when the surgeon encounters the situation of posteriorly dislocated lens fragments in conjunction with retinal breaks and a retinal detachment.[1,41] In the presence of a giant retinal tear or a large retinal dialysis, perfluorocarbon frequently becomes indispensable for a successful surgical outcome.[36] The retinal complications may be related to pre-existing retinal pathology, elicited by vitreoretinal traction associated with attempts to remove the lens fragments during the primary cataract surgery, or retinal injury from the dropped lens fragments subsequently.[1,5] The retinal breaks may also enlarge and a retinal detachment may progress during the process of lens fragment removal. In such a situation, perfluorocarbon liquid serves the dual purpose of stabilizing the retinal complications and preventing more retinal injury, while the lens fragments are floated anteriorly for phacoemulsification or removal through a limbal incision.[1,35,41] Any posterior hemorrhage from the retinal breaks may also be displaced anteriorly by the perfluorocarbon liquid for removal. With the retina held down by the perfluorocarbon liquid, standard vitreoretinal techniques are employed to repair the retinal breaks and detachment following the vitrectomy and elimination of the lens fragments. After the application of laser or cryotherapy and possible placement of a scleral buckle, fluid-air or gas exchange is performed to replace the perfluorocarbon liquid and to achieve appropriate retinal tamponade. In case of proliferative vitreoretinopathy, silicone oil may be required as the agent for prolonged retinal tamponade. Utilizing perfluorocarbon liquid in a manner similar to the above description, Lewis and others reported favorable outcome in managing dislocated lens fragments and IOLs.[41] Improved care and methods in the management of dislocated lens fragments during the primary cataract extraction and the subsequent surgery may be responsible for the much lower prevalence of associated retinal breaks and detachment in recent reports in contrast to earlier studies (3% to 5% versus 7% to 50%).[42] In a recent study, Moore and colleagues reported a combined incidence of 13.4% for retinal detachment associated with retained lens fragments and their subsequent surgical management (6.4% before pars plana vitrectomy and 7.0% after pars plana vitrectomy).[43]

CONCLUSION

Modern vitreoretinal surgery offers a variety of effective techniques in the safe removal of posteriorly dislocated lens fragments. Besides the standard 3-port pars plana vitrectomy with phacoemulsification, FAVIT is an expedient alternative for the cataract surgeon familiar with vitreoretinal techniques to promptly remove the lens fragments with minimal additional setup during the primary surgery. Perfluorocarbon liquid is a highly valuable intraoperative tool in managing the dislocated lens fragments and underlying associated retinal complications at the same time. Although cryoextraction provides a simple and direct means of removing a large and hard lens nucleus from the posterior segment, severe ocular complications may be associated with this technique. Its use should be limited to select cases by an experienced surgeon familiar with its potential hazards. Under the adverse condition of markedly poor visibility due to various causes, endoscopy can provide unparalleled viewing of the retro-irideal structures to allow safe removal of dislocated lens fragments irrespective of the degree of transparency of the anterior segment of the eye. Employing one or more of the techniques described in this chapter, favorable visual outcome can be achieved for the majority of eyes with dislocated lens fragments.

Key Points

- Small lens fragments consisting of mostly cortical material may gradually resolve with conservative medical management alone. However, large lens fragments with a sizeable nuclear component do not resolve and may elicit a phacoantigenic response from the host and so have to be removed.
- In the event of a rupture of the posterior lens capsule or zonular dehiscence leading to posterior migration of lens fragments, the cataract surgeon must avoid any uncontrolled and forceful surgical maneuvers in the vitreous cavity in an attempt to retrieve the sinking lens fragments.
- Any retrieval technique that does not provide for the appropriate management of the vitreous first has the potential of causing immediate or subsequent retinal complications.
- The cataract surgeon must refrain from the temptation of passing a sharp instrument or lens loop into the mid or posterior vitreous cavity to engage the sinking lens fragments, or passing forceful irrigation fluid into the vitreous cavity to float the lens fragments. Such maneuvers usually generate vitreoretinal traction resulting in retinal breaks and detachment.
- In case of familiarity with vitreoretinal techniques, one may convert over to a posterior segment setup and utilize one of the methods described

Contd...

Contd...

in the following sections for removing the lens fragments. Otherwise, a prompt referral of the patient to a vitreoretinal surgeon is recommended.
- Medical management with topical anti-inflammatory, antibiotic, as well as cycloplegic medications should be instituted. If necessary, hypotensive agents can also be utilized.
- Modern vitreoretinal surgery offers a variety of effective techniques in the safe removal of posteriorly dislocated lens fragments. Besides the standard 3-port pars plana vitrectomy with phacoemulsification, FAVIT is an expedient alternative for the cataract surgeon familiar with vitreoretinal techniques to promptly remove the lens fragments with minimal additional setup during the primary surgery.
- Use of Chandelier illumination helps one remove lens fragments by a true bimanual vitrectomy set up.
- Perfluorocarbon liquid is a highly valuable intraoperative tool in managing the dislocated lens fragments and underlying associated retinal complications at the same time.

REFERENCES

1. Chan CK, Lin SG. Management of dislocated lens and lens fragments by the vitreoretinal approach. In: Agarwal S, Agarwal A, Sachdev MS, et al. (eds). Phacoemulsification, Laser Cataract Surgery, and Foldable IOLs, 2nd edn. Jaypee Brothers Medical Publishers, Ltd, New Delhi. 2000.
2. Verhoeff FH, Lemoine AN. Endophthalmitis phacoanaphalactica. Am J Ophthalmol. 1922;5:737-61.
3. Apple DJ, Mamalis N, Steinmetz RI, et al. Phacoanaphylactic endophthalmitis associated with extracapsular cataract extraction and posterior chamber intraocular lens. Arch Ophthalmol. 1984;102:1528-32.
4. Smith RE, Weiner P. Unusual presentation of phacoanaphylaxis following phacoemulsification. Ophthalmic Surg. 1976;7:65-8.
5. Fastenberg DM, Schwartz PL, Shakin JL, et al. Management of dislocated nuclear fragments after phacoemulsification. Am J Ophthalmol. 1991;112:535-9.
6. Epstein DL. In: Chandler and Grant's glaucoma, 3rd edn. Lea and Febiger, Philadelphia. 1986:320-31.

7. Epstein DL. Diagnosis and management of lens-induced glaucoma. Ophthalmology. 1982;89:227-30.

8. Hutton WL, Snyder WB, Vaiser A. Management of surgically dislocated intravitreal lens fragments by pars plana vitrectomy. Ophthalmology. 1978;85:176-89.

9. Michels RG, Shacklett DE. Vitrectomy techniques for removal of retained lens material. Arch Ophthalmol. 1977;95:1767-73.

10. Ross WH. Management of dislocated lens fragments following phacoemulsification surgery. Can J Ophthalmol. 1993;28:163-6.

11. Blodi BA, Flynn HW Jr, Blodi CF, et al. Retained nuclei after cataract surgery. Ophthalmology. 1992;99:41-4.

12. Lambrou FH, Stewart MW. Management of dislocated lens fragments during phacoemulsification. Ophthalmology. 1992;99:1260-2.

13. Gilliland GD, Hutton WL, Fuller DG. Retained intravitreal lens fragments after cataract surgery. Ophthalmology. 1992;99:1263-7.

14. Kim JE, Flynn HW Jr, Smiddy WE, et al. Retained lens fragments after phacoemulsification. Ophthalmology. 1994;101:1827-32.

15. Verhoeff FH. A simple and safe method for removing a cataract dislocated into fluid vitreous. Am J Ophthalmol. 1942;25:725-6.

16. Charles S. Posterior dislocation of lens material during cataract surgery. In: Agarwal S, Agarwal A, Sachdev MS, et al (eds): Phacoemulsification, Laser Cataract Surgery, and Foldable IOLs, 2nd edn. Jaypee Brothers Medical Publishers, New Delhi. 2000. pp.517-21.

17. Topping TM. Management of dislocated lens fragments during phacoemulsification, and, Retained intravitreal lens fragments after cataract surgery [Discussion]. Ophthalmology. 1992;99:1268-9.

18. Gimbel HV, Penno EA. In: Agarwal S, Agarwal A. Sachdev MS, et al. (eds). Divide and Conquer Nucleofractis Techniques. 2nd edn. Jaypee Brothers Medical Publishers, New Delhi. 2000. pp.133-45.

19. Hara T. Endocapsular phacoemulsification and aspiration (ECPEA) – recent surgical technique and clinical results. Ophthalmic Surg. 1989;20:469-75.

20. Cionni RJ, Osher RH. Endocapsular ring approach to the subluxated cataractous lens. Cataract Refract Surg. 1995;21:245-9.

21. Eaton AM, Jaffe GJ, McCuen BW 2nd, et al. Condensation on the posterior surface of silicone intraocular lenses during fluid-air exchange. Ophthalmology. 1995;102:733-6.

22. Agarwal A, Narang P, Kumar DA, Agarwal A. Clinical outcomes of sleeveless phacotip assisted levitation of dropped nucleus. Br J

Ophthalmol. 2014 Feb 11. doi: 10.1136/bjophthalmol-2013-304737. [Epub ahead of print]

23. Elizalde J. Combined use of perfluorocarbon liquids and viscoelastics for safer surgical approach to posterior lens luxation. [Poster]. The Vitreous Society 17th Annual Meeting, Rome, Italy, September. 1999.pp.21-5.

24. Charles S. Vitreous microsurgery, 2nd edn, Williams and Wilkins, Baltimore. 1987. pp.48-51.

25. Ross WH. Management of dislocated lens fragments after phacoemulsification surgery. Can J Ophthalmol. 1996;31:234-40.

26. Eguchi S, Araie M. A new ophthalmic electronic videoendoscope system for intraocular surgery. Arch Ophthalmol. 1990;108:1778-81.

27. Grizzard WS. GRIN endoscopy. In syllabus: Subspecialty Day – Vitreoretinal Update, New Orleans. 1998.pp.109-12.

28. Uram M. Ophthalmic laser microendoscope endophotocoagulation. Ophthalmology. 1992;99:1829-32.

29. Uram M. Laser endoscope in the management of proliferative vitreoretinopathy. Ophthalmology. 1994;101:1404-8.

30. Fisher YL, Slakter JS. A disposable ophthalmic endoscopic system. Arch Ophthalmol. 1994;112:984-6.

31. Ciardella AP, Fisher YL, Carvalho C, et al. Endoscopic vitreoretinal surgery for complicated proliferative diabetic retinopathy. Retina. 2001;21:20-7.

32. Yaguchi S, Kora Y, Takahashi H, et al. A new endoscope for ophthalmic microsurgery. Ophthalmic Surg. 1992;23:838-41.

33. Boscher C, Lebuisson DA, Lean JS, et al. Vitrectomy with endoscopy for management of retained lens fragments and/or posteriorly dislocated intraocular lens. Graefes Arch Clin Exp Ophthalmol. 1998;236:115-21.

34. Barraquer J. Surgery of the dislocated lens. Trans Am Acad Ophthalmol Otolaryngol. 1975;76:44-9.

35. Shapiro MJ, Resnick KI, Kim SH, et al. Management of the dislocated crystalline lens with a perfluorocarbon liquid. Am J Ophthalmol. 1991;112:401-5.

36. Chang S. Perfluorocarbon liquids in vitreoretinal surgery. New approaches to vitreoretinal surgery. Int Ophthalmol Clin. 1992;32:153-63.

37. Rowson NJ, Bacon AS, Rosen PH. Perfluorocarbon heavy liquids in the management of posterior dislocation of the lens nucleus during phacoemulsification. Br J Ophthalmol. 1992;76:169-70.

38. Greve MD, Peyman GA, Mehta NJ, et al. Use of perfluoroperhydrophenanthrene in the management of posteriorly dislocated crystalline and intraocular lenses. Ophthalmic Surg. 1993;24:593-7.

39. Calhoun FP, Hagler WS. Experience with Jose Barraquer method of extracting a dislocated lens. Am J Ophthalmol. 1960;50:701-15.
40. Haymet BT. Removal of dislocated hypermature lens from the posterior vitreous. Aust NZJ Ophthalmol. 1990;18:103-6.
41. Lewis H, Blumenkranz MS, Chang S. Treatment of dislocated crystalline lens and retinal detachment with perfluorocarbon liquids. Retina. 1992;12:299-304.
42. Smiddy WE, Flynn HW Jr, Kim JE. Retinal detachment in patients with retained lens fragments or dislocated posterior chamber intraocular lenses. Ophthalmic Surg Lasers. 1996;27:856-61.
43. Moore JK, Scott IU, Flynn HW Jr, et al. Retinal detachment associated with retained lens fragments removed by pars plana vitrectomy [paper]. American Academy of Ophthalmology Annual Meeting, New Orleans, Louisiana, November 12. 2001.

10

Infectious Endophthalmitis

Clement K Chan, Steven G Lin

INTRODUCTION

Despite numerous recent advances in its treatment, infectious endophthalmitis continues to be one of the most serious complications in ophthalmology. The infectious organism associated with endophthalmitis causes prominent ocular inflammation and toxic reaction, leading to severe intraocular tissue damages and the consequential marked visual loss. Infectious endophthalmitis can be broadly divided into five types: 1) Acute or early-onset postoperative (usually after cataract extraction), 2) Chronic or late-onset, 3) Bleb-related, 4) Post-traumatic, and 5) Endogenous or metastatic. [1] The majority of endophthalmitis cases encountered by the practicing clinician consist of the first type: acute endophthalmitis after cataract extraction and intraocular lens (IOL) insertion.[1] However, any ocular surgery, including the relatively "nonpenetrating" ones (e.g. strabismus, refractive procedures, transscleral fixation of a posterior chamber implant-PCIOL) may result in endophthalmitis.[1-10]

CLINICAL FEATURES

The preliminary diagnosis of acute postoperative bacterial endophthalmitis must be based on clinical grounds alone, so that the clinician may initiate prompt intervention in time for an optimal outcome.[8,11] The classic presentation of acute postoperative bacterial endophthalmitis includes a red and painful eye associated with frequent headaches and prominent visual loss during the second to the seventh day after surgery.[1,11] The rapidly progressive symptoms are accompanied by diffuse lid and corneal edema, conjunctival discharge, as well as anterior chamber and vitreous infiltrates.[1,11] The increasing intraocular proteinaceous infiltrates frequently result in the layering of a fibrin clot within the bottom of the anterior chamber, known as a hypopyon.[11] Invasion of the retina and optic nerve by the infecting organism invariably leads to progressive disc and retinal edema and hemorrhage, posterior fibrin deposits, as well as tissue necrosis. The eventual severe retinal destruction results in profound visual loss. The necrotic retina is also prone to develop retinal breaks and detachments during and subsequent to the course of the endophthalmitis.[12] Whether other clinical features are present or not, the cardinal sign and the only consistent and reliable indicator of postoperative endophthalmitis is unexplained vitreous inflammation and opacification.[8] In the endophthalmitis vitrectomy study (EVS), pain was absent in 25% of cases and hypopyon was lacking in 14% of cases.[8,13] Typical clinical signs may also be masked and their onset delayed on account of postoperative antibiotic and corticosteroid usage, as well as the low virulence of the causative organism.[1,14,15]

Organisms Associated with Acute Postoperative Endophthalmitis

The most common microbial isolate from acute postoperative endophthalmitis is a gram-positive organism; specifically, a coagulase-negative *Staphylococcus*.[1,15-18] The EVS reported 70% of the isolates to be coagulase-negative micrococci (predominantly staphylococci).[18] Twenty-four point two (24.2%) of the isolates consisted of other gram-positive organisms as follow: 9.9% *Staphylococcus aureus*, 9.0% *Streptococcus* species, 2.2% *Enterococcus* species, and 3.1% miscellaneous gram-positive species (0.6% *Propionibacterium* species, 1.2% *Corynebacterium* species, 0.6% *Bacillus* species, and 0.6% *Diphtheroid*.)[18] Gram- negative organisms were isolated in 5.9% of the cases in the EVS (1.9% *Proteus mirabilis*, 1.2% *Pseudomonas* species, 0.6% *Morganella morganii*, 0.6% *Citrobacter diversus*, 0.3% *Serratia marcescens*, 0.6% *Enterobacter* species, and 0.3% *Flavobacterium* species).[18-50] It is possible that the EVS may have underestimated the rate of gram-negative infection for postoperative endophthalmitis by excluding eyes with corneal opacities severe enough to preclude a vitrectomy.[8] Table 10.1 outlines a typical spectrum of microbial isolates associated with acute postoperative endophthalmitis (reported in the EVS), as well as distinctive spectra of microbial isolates associated with other types of endophthalmitis.[1,6,16-18,36,41-46,49]

Delayed-onset Endophthalmitis

Chronic or late-onset endophthalmitis is defined as the presentation of indolent intraocular inflammation one or more months after ocular surgery. Traditionally, fungal endophthalmitis has often been cited as an example of late-onset endophthalmitis.[1,11,19] However, recent reports have also implicated other organisms associated with this category of endophthalmitis.[20-27] In their review of 19 cases of delayed-onset pseudophakic endophthalmitis, Fox and associates reported 63% of those cases to be due to *Propionibacterium acnes*, 16% to *Candida parapsilosis*, 16% to *Staphylococcus epidermidis*, and 5% to *Corynebacterium* species.[26] Ficker et al. isolated *Staphylococcus epidermidis* and *Achromobacter* species from eyes with chronic bacterial endophthalmitis.[27]

Propionibacterium Endophthalmitis

In 1986, Meister and associates described the syndrome of *Propionibacterium acnes* endophthalmitis with delayed onset after

TABLE 10.1 Protocol for intravitreal antibiotic preparation

Vancomycin hydrochloride: 1 mg in 0.1 mL
- Add 10 mL of diluent to 500 mg powder in vial, resulting in 50 mg/mL concentration
- Insert 2 mL (100 mg) or reconstituted drug into 10 mL sterile empty vial, and add 8 mL of diluent, resulting in a final solution of **10 mg/mL***

Ceftazidime hydrochloride: 2.25 mg in 0.1 mL
- Add 10 mL of diluent to 500 mg powder in vial to result in 50 mg/mL concentration
- Insert 1 mL (50 mg) of reconstituted drug into a 10 mL sterile empty vial, and mix with 1.2 mL of diluent, for a final solution of **22.5 mg/mL***

Cefazolin sodium: 2.25 mg in 0.1 mL
- Add 2 mL of diluent to 500 mg powder in vial to result in concentration of 225 mg/mL
- Insert 1 mL (22.5 mg) of reconstituted drug into a 10 mL sterile empty vial, and mix with additional 9 mL of diluent, for a final solution of **22.5 mg/mL***

Amikacin sulfate: 0.2 to 0.4 mg in 0.1 mL
- Original vial contains 500 mg in 2 mL (250 mg/mL) solution
- Add 0.8 mL (200 mg) solution into a 10 mL sterile empty vial, and mix with additional 9.2 mL of diluent, to achieve a concentration of 200 mg in 10 mL (20 mg/mL)
- Withdraw 0.2 mL (4 mg) and mix with 0.8 mL of diluent in a second sterile empty vial to achieve final solution of **0.4 mg/mL**;* or withdraw 0.1 mL (2 mg) and mix with 0.9 mL of diluent to achieve a final solution of **0.2 mg/mL***

Gentamicin sulfate: 0.1 to 0.2 mg in 0.1 mL
- Original vial contains 80 mg in 2 mL (40 mg/mL) solution
- Add 0.1 mL (4 mg) solution into a 10 mL sterile empty vial, and mix with 3.9 mL of diluent to achieve a solution of 4 mg in 4 mL or **1 mg/1 mL**;* or add 0.2 mL (8 mg) solution into a 10 mL sterile empty vial, and mix with 3.9 mL of diluent to achieve a solution of 8 mg in 4 mL or **2 mg/1 mL***

Clindamycin phosphate: 1 mg in 0.1 mL
- Original vial contains a 600 mg in 4 mL solution (15 0 mg/1 mL)
- Add 0.2 mL (30 mg) solution into a 10 mL sterile empty vial and mix with 2.8 mL of diluent to achieve a solution of 30 mg in 3 mL or **10 mg/mL***

Contd...

Contd...

Chloramphenicol sodium succinate: 2 mg in 0.1 mL
- Original vial contains 1000 mg powder.
- Add 10 mL of diluent to reconstitute 1000 mg powder for a concentration of 100 mg/mL.
- Withdraw 1 mL of reconstituted drug (100 mg) and mix with 4 mL of diluent in a 10 mL sterile empty vial to achieve a final solution of **20 mg/1 mL**.*

Amphotericin B: 0.005 mg in 0.1 mL
- Original vial contains 50 mg powder
- Add 10 mL of diluent to reconstitute the 50 mg powder into a concentration of 5 mg/mL
- Add 0.1 mL (0.5 mg) of reconstituted solution into a 10 mL sterile empty vial, and mix with 9.9 mL of diluent to achieve a final solution of **0.05 mg/1 mL***

Miconazole: 0.025 mg in 0.1 mL
- Original ampule contains 20 mL of 10 mg/mL solution
- Remove glass particles and impurities by passing solution into a 5-μm filter needle
- Add 0.25 mL (2.5 mg) of filtered solution into a 10 mL sterile empty vial, and mix with 9.75 mL of diluent to achieve a final solution of 2.5 mg in 10 mL or **0.25 mg/1 mL***

Recommendation: For optimal results, the drug dilution and preparation should be performed by trained personnel in the controlled environment of a hospital pharmacy.[1,107] Nonbacteriostatic sterile water is used as diluent for vancomycin and amphotericin B. For all others, nonbacteriostatic sterile water or 0.9 % sodium chloride solution is used as diluent.[1,108] * For all medications, the volume from the final solution for intravitreal injection is 0.1 mL drawn into a tuberculin syringe and delivered with a 27- or 30-gauge needle at the pars plana.[1,108]

---

extracapsular cataract extraction (ECCE) with posterior chamber intraocular lens (PCIOL) implantation.[20] *Propionibacterium* is a gram-positive, nonspore-forming, pleomorphic and anaerobic bacillus. It is ubiquitous in nature and a common component of the bacterial flora of the ocular and periocular tissues, including the conjunctiva and the sebaceous follicles.[20,32] It is an opportunistic pathogen frequently associated with a low-grade, delayed-onset, and persistent endophthalmitis after cataract extraction with an intraocular implant.[20-26] The typical clinical presentation may include an indolent course of chronic low-grade iridocyclitis with one or more of the following signs—large white granulomatous or nongranulomatous keratic precipitates, hypopyon, beaded fibrin strands in the anterior chamber, vitritis, intraretinal hemorrhages and infiltrates, and a prominent whitish plaque on the residual lens capsule.[20-26] The last feature is considered to be a hallmark sign of *P. acnes* endophthalmitis.[25,32] Previous biopsies of lens capsules with the whitish exudates have yielded *P. acnes* on histological studies and cultures, proving that they contain foci of sequestered *P. acnes* organisms.[21-25,32] The delayed activation and proliferation of the sequestered organisms result in a chronic and indolent course of endophthalmitis.[51-80] Since *P. acnes* is a low virulent and fastidious bacillus, it is difficult to isolate and grow in culture.[20] Specimens of suspected cases of *P. acnes* endophthalmitis should be promptly inoculated into anaerobic media. *P. acnes* may not appear in culture until 5 days or more after inoculation.[20] It has been pointed out that the *P. acnes* organisms isolated from eyes with acute postoperative endophthalmitis may constitute a less resilient form than those from eyes with the delayed-onset or chronic type of endophthalmitis.[33] Unlike the chronic *P. acnes* infection, the acute type is usually easily eradicated with intravitreal antibiotic injections alone and has a low recurrence rate.[1,33] In contrast, the chronic *P. acnes* endophthalmitis frequently requires a vitrectomy and capsulectomy to eliminate the sequestered organisms.[20,25,32]

DIAGNOSTIC WORKUP AND MICROBIOLOGICAL STUDIES

When managing an eye with suspected endophthalmitis, the clinician must first perform a careful evaluation. It is important to pay close attention to certain ocular features that may modify the course and influence the management of the infection, e.g. wound leak and dehiscence, iris and vitreous prolapse, flat anterior chamber, corneal and suture abscess, bleb defects, eroding scleral suture associated with a sutured posterior chamber implant, etc.[1,8] A successful outcome entails the correction of the above abnormalities besides effective antimicrobial therapy. One must also differentiate endophthalmitis from other conditions with similar clinical features, such as a corneal ulcer and aseptic anterior uveitis with a hypopyon, and vitreous infiltration due to sterile posterior uveitis or retained lens fragments, phacoanaphylactic uveitis, etc. In addition, a search for concomitant conditions that may complicate the course of the endophthalmitis is an important part of the workup, e.g. superimposed retinal breaks or detachment, choroidal detachment, located lens fragments, and intraocular foreign body, etc. Ancillary diagnostic tools such as ultrasonography may contribute to the diagnostic workup.[1,8]

Techniques of Specimen Collection

Aqueous and vitreous specimens may be obtained in an office setting or at the time of a vitrectomy. In the former situation, careful administration of local anesthesia (topical, subconjunctival, peribulbar, or retrobulbar) and sterile prepping with 5% povidone-iodine solution are recommended.[1,8,13,81] A small volume of aqueous specimen (0.1–0.2 mL) is then carefully withdrawn via a 27- or 30-gauge needle at the limbus into a tuberculin syringe. The vitreous specimen may be obtained with one of the following two methods: [8,13,81]

Needle Tap

A 22- to 27- gauge needle attached to a tuberculin syringe is inserted through the pars plana into the vitreous cavity for gentle aspiration of 0.1 to 0.3 mL of liquid vitreous. Excessive force must be avoided to prevent vitreoretinal traction. A "dry tap" requires the conversion to a mechanized biopsy.

Mechanized Vitreous Biopsy

A one-, two-, or three-port pars plana vitrectomy with a mechanized 20-gauge vitrectomy probe is employed for the biopsy. A small volume of undiluted specimen (up to 0.3 mL) from the anterior vitreous is collected into a sterile syringe connected to the aspiration

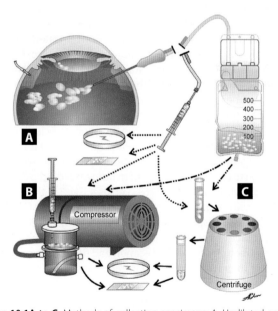

Figures 10.1A to C Methods of collecting specimens: A. Undiluted aqueous and vitreous specimens may be directly inoculated onto culture media and used for smear preparation; B. Diluted vitreous specimen collected into a syringe or a cassette is either first concentrated by vacuuming the diluted fluid in a sterile upper chamber through a 0.45-μm membrane filter into a lower sterile chamber (suction filter method); C. Concentrated in a sterile centrifuge tube after performing high-speed centrifuge (centrifuge method). Small cut segments of the membrane filter with the concentrated specimens or the sediments from the centrifuged tube are innoculated into culture media and applied on slides for smear preparation

line of the vitrectomy probe through gentle manual suction by a surgical assistant during the vitrectomy. Diluted specimens collected into a larger syringe or into a vitrectomy cassette may also be concentrated either with the suction filtered technique or the centrifuged method (Figs 10.1A to C).[1,8,82,83] The former involves passing the diluted specimens in an upper sterile chamber through a membrane filter with 0.45-micron pores into a lower chamber connected to suction. With the aid of sterile forceps and scissors or knives, the membrane filter containing the concentrated specimens is then cut into small pieces for direct inoculation on solid and into liquid media for cultures (Fig. 10.1).[1,82] Concentrated specimens scraped off the surface of the membrane filter are also applied on slides for preparation of various stains. The alternative centrifuged method requires the transfer of the diluted specimens into a sterile centrifuge tube for high-speed centrifuge. The sediments from the centrifuged tube are then processed for microbiological stains and cultures (Fig. 10.1). In 1993, Donahue and associates reported a significant increase in positive yield with culturing the contents of a vitrectomy cassette after concentration of the specimen in comparison to culturing the specimen from a needle tap or a limited mechanized vitreous biopsy (76% versus 43%).[83] In the EVS, some degree of culture growth was achieved from 82.8% of the tested vitrectomy cassette specimens, and the vitrectomy cassette fluid was the only source of a positive culture for 8.9% of eyes.[81] The EVS found that the vitrectomy cassette specimen had prognostic significance equivalent to growth from other intraocular sources.[84-86]

TREATMENT OF ENDOPHTHALMITIS

The two fundamental therapeutic modalities for treating infectious endophthalmitis in the modern world comprise of antimicrobial therapy and vitrectomy. When appropriate, they may be supplemented with anti-inflammatory therapy for reducing damages induced by the infection. Applying effective strategies for antimicrobial therapy constitutes the most critical aspect of the management of endophthalmitis.

Antimicrobial Therapy

Topical and Subconjunctival

Prophylactic therapy: Multiple studies have demonstrated that preoperative application of antiseptics and antibiotics with a broad-spectrum antimicrobial coverage reduces the eyelid and conjunctival bacterial counts, resulting in decreased potential for postoperative endophthalmitis.[87-90] Apt and associates reported that a single preoperative application of half-strength (5%) povidone-iodine solution in the conjunctival cul-de-sac was equivalent to a 3-day course of prophylactic topical combination solution of neomycin sulfate, polymyxin B sulfate, and gramicidin in reducing the bacterial colonies.[87-89]

Therapy after the onset of endophthalmitis: With the exception of mild infections, topical and subconjunctival drug delivery usually constitutes only adjunctive antimicrobial therapy after the onset of endophthalmitis. However, they are essential for certain conditions that may accompany the endophthalmitis (i.e. bleb infection, corneal ulcer, wound or suture abscess, etc.)[1,8] A typical regimen of supplemental topical therapy for acute postoperative bacterial endophthalmitis includes frequent application of antibiotics with appropriate antibacterial coverage, as well as repeated administration of anti-inflammatory and cycloplegic drugs.[91-110] Steroid is avoided for fungal cases. The use of customized fortified doses of topical antimicrobial drugs (e.g. 45 to 50 mg/mL of vancomycin, 50 mg/mL of cefazolin, cefamandole or ceftazidime, 50 mg/mL of ampicillin, 50 mg/mL of clindamycin, 1% solution of methicillin, 8 to 15 mg/mL of tobramycin, 10 to 20 mg/mL of gentamicin or amikacin, 0.15 to 0.5% of amphotericin B, or 10 mg/mL of miconazole, etc.) has been a common practice in the course of treating the endophthalmitis.[8,13] However, the potential benefit of the fortified doses over the regular doses remains controversial and unproven. Another common practice is supplemental subconjunctival therapy (e.g. 25 mg of vancomycin, 100 to 125 mg of cefazolin, or ceftazidime, 75 mg of cefamandole, 100 mg of ampicillin or methicillin, 20 to 40 mg of gentamicin, tobramycin or amikacin, 30 mg of clindamycin, or 5 mg of miconazole.)[1,8,13] The degree of synergy between subconjunctival and intravitreal antimicrobial therapy is unknown.

Intravitreal Antimicrobial Therapy

For all categories of endophthalmitis besides the endogenous type, the mainstay of therapy is prompt and direct intravitreal injections of antimicrobial drugs.[1,8] It is imperative that the intravitreal antimicrobial therapy first provides comprehensive coverage for the gram-positive organisms, since they constitute the majority of the microbial isolates associated with endophthalmitis (94% in the EVS).[1,8,18]

The following antibiotic combinations are the current recommended initial empiric intravitreal antibiotic regimens for acute postoperative bacterial endophthalmitis in a clinical setting:[1,8,13]

- Vancomycin 1.0 mg/0.1 mL and ceftazidime 2.25 mg/0.1 mL; or
- Vancomycin 1.0 mg/0.1 mL and amikacin (100 to 400 μg/0.1 mL) for beta-lactam sensitive patients.

Table 10.1 provides detailed protocol for the preparation and dosages of commonly used intraocular drugs for endophthalmitis.

Systemic Antimicrobial Therapy

Although the EVS found systemic antimicrobial therapy provide no additional benefit to intravitreal therapy for acute postoperative endophthalmitis, its role for other types of endophthalmitis is more important.[13,111] Concomitant intravitreal and systemic antibiotic therapy besides vitrectomy remains to be the standard of care (based on clinical experience but without experimental support) for most bleb-related and trauma-induced endophthalmitis.[34,36,41,111-116] For endogenous endophthalmitis, appropriate systemic (especially intravenous) therapy with maximal doses for intravitreal penetration is the key for a successful outcome.[49,111] Intravenous antibiotic therapy is generally required for two weeks for most endogenous cases, and as long as four or more weeks for endocarditis cases.[50]

Corticosteroid therapy

The use of intravitreal corticosteroids for non-fungal endophthalmitis remains controversial due to a lack of randomized controlled studies.[8,117] The potential benefits of corticosteroid therapy for endophthalmitis include inhibition of macrophage and neutrophil migration, stabilization of lysosomal membranes resulting in decreased degranulation of inflammatory cells (neutrophils, mast cells, macrophages, basophils), and reduction in prostaglandin synthesis and capillary permeability due to inhibition of phospholipase A_2.[117] However, its potential harmful effects and limitations include possible reduction in the killing power of inflammatory cells, changes in the bioavailability and doses of the intravitreal antibiotics, potentiation of the infection in the absence of appropriate antibiotic therapy, risk of retinal toxicity due to medication errors, and inability to counteract bacterial toxin-induced damages.[117] The standard clinical dose of intravitreal dexamethasone is 400 µg/0.1 mL,[118-124] although the optimal dose has not been determined.[1,8,125-128] Besides intravitreal injections, other routes of steroid therapy include subconjunctival injections (4 to 12 mg of dexamethasone or 40 mg of triamcinolone or depomedrol) and systemic therapy (1 mg/kg/day for 5 days followed by rapid tapering).[8,13,117] When fungal endophthalmitis is suspected, most authorities advocate the avoidance of corticosteroid.[129-149]

Vitrectomy

Indications for Vitrectomy

The theoretical advantages of vitrectomy include the removal of infectious organisms with their toxins and inflammatory mediators, clearing of vitreous opacities and sequestered abscess pockets, collection of abundant specimens for cultures, elimination of vitreous membranes to avoid vitreoretinal traction, allowing increased space for intraocular drug administration, and possible improved diffusion of intravitreal antibiotics.[1,13] For chronic endophthalmitis due to the *Propionibacterium* species, intravitreal antibiotics alone may not be sufficient. Frequently, a vitrectomy combined with a partial or complete removal of the lens capsule with sequestered organisms (sometimes including the implant), is required for a successful outcome.[20,23,25,26,32]

Vitrectomy Techniques

A three-port pars plana vitrectomy using standard 20-gauge instruments and concentrating on the "core" vitreous is usually recommended, although a one- or two-port approach may be sufficient for a limited vitreous biopsy.[8] A portable battery-driven 23-gauge vitrector is also commercially available for a limited vitreous biopsy.[8] The greater potential for surgical complications associated with increased tissue vulnerability induced by the endophthalmitis requires the surgeon to be well versed with vitreoretinal techniques and vigilant throughout the vitrectomy. The use of a long infusion cannula (e.g. 6 mm) is often advantageous in preventing subretinal and choroidal infusion for pseudophakic eyes and post-traumatic eyes requiring a lensectomy, in light of multiple predisposing factors for such a complication with endophthalmitis (e.g. limited intraocular tissue visibility, increased choroidal congestion, frequent hypotony, etc.) To further avoid such a complication, the surgeon must ensure that the tip of the infusion cannula is well within the vitreous cavity before turning on the infusion fluid. For a case with very cloudy media, the surgeon may confirm this by gently rubbing the tip of a microvitreoretinal blade inserted through one of the superior sclerotomies against the tip of the infusion cannula. Frequently, a separate anterior chamber washout via a limbal approach is required to eliminate cloudy fibrin deposits and hyphema from the anterior chamber initially, before sufficient anterior media clarity is attained for a pars plana vitrectomy. Various microsurgical hooks and picks may be inserted through the limbus to scrape off the anterior chamber infiltrates or membranes layered on the surface of the implant and the iris before removing them with a vitrectomy probe from the

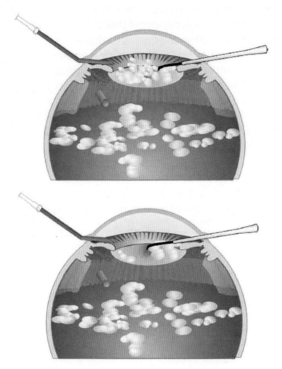

Figure 10.2 Anterior chamber washout before vitrectomy: The technique of eliminating cloudy fibrin deposits, membranes, and hyphema from the anterior chamber is illustrated. A microsurgical hook or pick inserted at the limbus is used to scrape off the cloudy material from the IOL and iris surface before removing them with a vitrectomy probe from the anterior chamber. A separate probe also inserted at the limbus for anterior chamber infusion is often necessary to prevent chamber collapse. The posterior infusion fluid is not turned on until adequate media clarity is achieved to ascertain the proper location of the tip of the posterior infusion cannula

anterior chamber (Fig. 10.2). A separate anterior infusion line may be required during the anterior chamber washout to prevent chamber collapse. When performing a core vitrectomy, care must be taken to apply only gentle intraocular movements and avoid vigorous surgical maneuvers that may induce vitreoretinal traction, such as aggressive epiretinal membrane retrieval and fibrin clean up. Despite the intentional avoidance of their direct removal during the vitrectomy, the posterior epiretinal fibrin deposits and dense retinal hemorrhages tend to gradually dissolve following the injections of intravitreal antimicrobial and anti-inflammatory medications after surgery. Keeping the intraocular instruments well within the anterior and central vitreous cavity and staying away from the fragile infected retina during surgery, will reduce the chance of retinal complications. Vitreous specimen for microbial investigation is either collected into a syringe connected to the aspiration line of the vitrectomy probe or into a cassette of the vitrectomy machine (Fig. 10.1).[8] Finally, the eye is made sufficiently soft to allow space for injections of medications and the sclerotomies are closed tightly to avoid fluid leaks, before the administration of intravitreal drugs at the end of the surgery.

CONCLUSION

Highly effective therapy is available for treating infectious endophthalmitis in the twenty-first century. Empiric intravitreal antimicrobial regimens in a "shot gun" approach constitute the first line of therapy with a proven track record in treating most forms of endophthalmitis. New advances in antimicrobial therapy allow consistent control of infections induced by a broad spectrum of organisms.

Key Points

- The infectious organism associated with endophthalmitis causes prominent ocular inflammation and toxic reaction, leading to severe intraocular tissue damages and the consequential marked visual loss.
- The classic presentation of acute postoperative bacterial endophthalmitis includes a red and painful eye associated with frequent headaches and prominent visual loss during the second to the seventh day after surgery.
- Chronic or late-onset endophthalmitis is defined as the presentation of indolent intraocular inflammation one or more months after ocular surgery.
- *Propionibacterium* is a gram-positive, nonspore-forming, pleomorphic and anaerobic bacillus. It is ubiquitous in nature and a common component of the bacterial flora of the ocular and periocular tissues, including the conjunctiva and the sebaceous follicles.
- Aqueous and vitreous specimens may be obtained in an office setting or at the time of a vitrectomy.
- The two fundamental therapeutic modalities for treating infectious endophthalmitis in the modern world comprise of antimicrobial therapy and vitrectomy.

REFERENCES

1. Forster RK. Endophthalmitis. In: Tasman W, Jaeger EA (eds): Duane's Clinical Ophthalmology. Philadelphia, Lippincott-Raven. 1996;4(24):1-29.
2. Heilskov T, Joondeph BC, Olsen KR, et al. Case report: Late endophthalmitis after transscleral fixation of a posterior chamber intraocular lens. Arch Ophthalmol. 1989;107:1427.
3. Christy NE, Lall P. Postoperative endophthalmitis following cataract surgery. Arch Ophthalmol. 1973;90:361-6.
4. Kattan HM, Flynn HW Jr, Pflugfelder S, et al. Nosocomial endophthalmitis survey. Ophthalmology. 1991;98:227-38.
5. Leveille AS, McMullan FD, Cavanagh HD. Endophthalmitis following penetrating keratoplasty. Ophthalmology. 1983;90:38-9.
6. Brinton GS, Topping TM, Hyndiuk RA, et al. Posttraumatic endophthalmitis. Arch Ophthalmol. 1984;102:547-50.

7. Boldt HC, Pulido JS, Blodi CF, et al. Rural endophthalmitis. Ophthalmology. 1989;96:1722-6.

8. Han DP. Acute-onset postoperative endophthalmitis: Current recommendations. In syllabus: Subspecialty Day-Retina, Management of posterior segment complications of anterior segment surgery. 1998.

9. Starr MB. Prophylactic antibiotics for ophthalmic surgery. Surv Ophthalmol. 1983;27:353-73.

10. Javitt JC, Vitale S, Canner JK, et al. National outcomes of cataract extraction. Arch Ophthalmol. 1991;109:1085-9.

11. Wilson FM, Wilson II FM. Postoperataive uveitis. In: Tasman W, Jaeger EA (eds). Duane's Clinical Ophthalmology. Philadelphia, Lippincott-Raven. 1996;4(55):1-18.

12. Nelson PT, Marcus DA, Bovino JA. Retinal detachment following endophthalmitis. Ophthalmology. 1985;92:1112-7.

13. Endophthalmitis Vitrectomy Study Group. Results of the Endophthalmitis Vitrectomy Study. A randomized trial of immediate vitrectomy and intravenous antibiotics for the treatment of postoperative bacterial endophthalmitis. Arch Ophthalmol. 1995;113:1479-96.

14. Bode DD, Gelender H, Forster RK. A retrospective review of endophthalmitis due to coagulase-negative staphylococci. Br J Ophthalmol. 1985;69:915-9.

15. Ormerod LD, Ho DD, Becker LE, et al. Endophthalmitis caused by the coagulase-negative staphylococci: I. Disease spectrum and outcome. Ophthalmology. 1993;100:715-23.

16. Forster RK, Abbott RL, Gelender H. Management of infectious endophthalmitis. Ophthalmology. 1980;87:313-9.

17. Puliafito CA, Baker AS, Haaf J, et al. Infectious endophthalmitis. Ophthalmology. 1982;89:921-9.

18. Han DP, Wisniewski SR, Wilson LA, et al. Spectrum and susceptibilities of microbiologic isolates in the Endophthalmitis Vitrectomy Study. Am J Ophthalmol. 1996;112:1-17.

19. Theodore FH. Symposium: Postoperative endophthalmitis; Etiology and diagnosis of fungal postoperative endophthalmitis. Ophthalmology. 1978;85:327-40.

20. Meisler DM, Palestine AG, Vastine DW, et al. Chronic *Propionibacterium* endophthalmitis after cataract extraction and intraocular lens implantation. Am J Ophthalmol. 1986;102:733-9.

21. Jaffe GJ, Whitcher JP, Biswell R, et al. Propionibacterium acnes endophthalmitis seven months after extracapsular cataract extraction and intraocular lens implantation. Ophthalmic Surg. 1986;17:791-3.

22. Roussel TJ, Culbertson WW, Jaffe NS. Chronic postoperative endophthalmitis associated with *Propionibacterium acnes*. Arch Ophthalmol. 1987;105:1199-201.

23. Meisler DM, Zakov ZN, Bruner WE, et al. Endophthalmitis associated with sequestered intraocular *Propionibacterium acnes* [letter]. Am J Ophthalmol. 1987;104:428-9.

24. Brady SE, Cohen EJ, Fischer DH. Diagnosis and treatment of chronic postoperative bacterial endophthalmitis. Ophthalmic Surg. 1988;19:580-4.

25. Meisler DM, Mandelbaum S. Propionibacterium-associated endophthalmitis after extracapsular cataract extraction. Review of reported cases. Ophthalmology. 1989;96:54-61.

26. Fox GM, Joondeph BC, Flynn HW Jr, et al. Delayed-onset pseudophakic endophthalmitis. Am J Ophthalmol. 1991;111:163-73.

27. Ficker L, Meredith TA, Wilson LA, et al. Chronic bacterial endophthalmitis. Am J Ophthalmol. 1987;103:745-8.

28. Roussel TJ, Olson ER, Rice T, et al. Chronic postoperative endoph-thalmitis associated with *Actinomyces* species. Arch Ophthalmol. 1991;109:60-2.

29. Zimmerman PL, Mamalis N, Alder JB, et al. Chronic Nocardia asteroides endophthalmitis after extracapsular cataract extraction. Arch Ophthalmol. 1993;111:837-40.

30. Pettit TH, Olson RJ, Foos RY, et al. Fungal endophthalmitis following intraocular lens implantation. Arch Ophthalmol. 1980;98:1025-39.

31. Stern WH, Tamura E, Jacobs RA, et al. Epidemic post-surgical *Candida parapsilosis* endophthalmitis. Ophthalmology. 1985;92:1701-9.

32. Zambrano W, Flynn HW Jr, Pflugfelder SC, et al. Management options for *Propionibacterium acnes* endophthalmitis. Ophthalmology. 1989;96:1100-5.

33. Winward KE, Pflugfelder SC, Flynn HW Jr, et al. Postoperative *Propionibacterium* endophthalmitis. Ophthalmology. 1993;100:447-51.

34. Ciulla TA, Beck AD, Topping TM, et al. Blebitis, early endophthalmitis, and late endophthalmitis after glaucoma-filtering surgery. Ophthalmology. 1997;104:986-95.

35. Brown RH, Yang LH, Walker SD, et al. Treatment of bleb infection after glaucoma surgery. Arch Ophthalmol. 1994;112:57-61.

36. Mandelbaum S, Forster RK, Gelender H et al. Late onset endophthalmitis associated with filtering blebs. Ophthalmology. 1985;92:964-72.

37. Parrish R, Minckler D. Late endophthalmitis: Filtering surgery time bomb? [editorial]. Ophthalmology. 1996;103:1167-8.

38. Wolner B, Liebermann JM, Sassan JW, et al. Late bleb-related endophthalmitis after trabeculectomy with adjunctive 5-fluorouracil. Ophthalmology. 1991;98:1053-60.

39. Higginbotham EJ, Stevens RK, Musch D, et al. Bleb-related endophthalmitis after trabeculectomy with mitomycin C. Ophthalmology. 1996;103:650-6.

40. Jett BD, Jensen HG, Atkuri RV, et al. Evaluation of therapeutic measures for treating endophthalmitis caused by isogenic toxin producing and toxin- nonproducing *Enterococcus faecalis* strains. Invest Ophthalmol Vis Sci. 1995;36:9-15.

41. Parrish CM, O'Day D. Traumatic endophthalmitis. Int Ophthalmol Clin. 1987;27:112-119.

42. Bohigan GM, Olk RJ. Factors associated with a poor visual result in endophthalmitis. Am J Ophthalmol. 1986;101:332-4.

43. Schemmer GB, Driebe WT. Posttraumatic *Bacillus cereus* endophthalmitis. Arch Ophthalmol. 1987;105:342-4.

44. Rowsey JJ, Newsom DL, Sexton DJ, et al. Endophthalmitis, current approaches. Ophthalmology. 1982;89:1055-66.

45. Affeldt JC, Flynn HW, Forster RK, et al. Ophthalmology. 1987;94:407-13.

46. Peyman GA, Raichand M, Bennett TO, et al. Management of endophthalmitis with pars plana vitrectomy. Br J Ophthalmol. 1980;64:472-5.

47. O'Day, Smith RS, Gregg CR. The problem of Bacillus species infection with special emphasis on the virulence of Bacillus cereus. Ophthalmology. 1981;88:833-8.

48. Bouza E, Grant S, Jordan MC, et al. Bacillus cereus endogenous panophthalmitis. Arch Ophthalmol. 1979;97:498-9.

49. Greenwald MJ, Wohl LG, Sell CH. Metastatic bacterial endophthalmitis: A contemporary reappraisal. Surv Ophthalmol. 1986;31:81-101.

50. Okada AA, Johnson P, Liles C, et al. Endogenous bacterial endophthalmitis. Ophthalmology. 1994;101:832-8.

51. Farber BP, Weinbaum DL, Dummer JS. Metastatic bacterial endophthalmitis. Arch Intern Med. 1985;145:62-4.

52. Reed M, Hibberd PL. Endoscopy and endophthalmitis [letter]. N Engl J Med. 1989;321:836.

53. Sugar HS, Mandell GH, Shalev J. Metastatic endophthalmitis associated with injection of addictive drugs. Am J Ophthalmol. 1971;71:1055-8.

54. Michelson JB, Friedlaender MH. Endophthalmitis of drug abuse. Int Ophthalmol Clin. 1987;27:120-6.

55. Clarkson JG, Green WR. Endogenous fungal endophthalmitis. In: Duane ET (ed): Duane's Clinical Ophthalmology. Hagerstown, MD, Harper and Row. 1976;3(11).

56. Aziz AA, Bullock JD, Mcguire TW, et al. Aspergillus endophthalmitis: A clinical and experimental study. Trans Am Ophthalmol Soc. 1992;90:317-42, discussion 342-6.

57. Doft BH, Clarkson JG, Rebell G, et al. Endogenous Aspergillus endophthalmitis in drug abusers. Arch Ophthalmol. 1980;98:859-62.

58. Diamond JG. Intraocular management of endophthalmitis. A systematic approach. Arch Ophthalmol. 1981;99:96-9.

59. Lewis PM. Ocular complications of meningococcic meningitis: Observations in 350 cases. Am J Ophthalmol. 1940;23:617-32.

60. Frantz JF, Lemp MA, Font RL, et al. Acute endogenous panophthalmitis caused by *Clostridium perfringens*. Am J Ophthalmol. 1974;78:295-303.

61. Abbott RL, Forster RK, Rebell G. Listeria monocytogenes endophthalmitis with a black hypopyon. Am J Ophthalmol. 1978;86:715-9.

62. Ballan PH, Loffredo FR, Painter B. *Listeria endophthalmitis*. Arch Ophthalmol. 1979;97:101-2.

63. Taylor JRW, Cibis GW, Hamtil LW. Endophthalmitis complicating *Haemophilis influenzae* type B meningitis. Arch Ophthalmol. 1980;98:324-6.

64. Boomla K, Quilliam RP. *Haemophilis influenzae* endophthalmitis. Br Med J. 1981;282:989-90.

65. Shammas HF. Endogenous *E. coli* endophthalmitis. Surv Ophthalmol. 1977;21:429-35.

66. Cohen P, Kirshner J, Whiting G. Bilateral endogenous *Escherichia coli* endophthalmitis. Arch Intern Med. 1980;140:1088-9.
67. Malan P, Zaluski S, Boudet C. Endophthalmic endogene bilaterale a klebsiella. Bull soc Ophthalmol Fr. 1984;84:961-4.
68. Sipperly JO, Shore JW. Septic retinal cyst in endogenous *Klebsiella* endophthalmitis. Am J Ophthalmol. 1982;94:124-5.
69. Gammon JA, Schwab I, Joseph P. Gentamicin-resistant Serratia marcescens endophthalmitis. Arch Ophthalmol. 1980;98:1221-23.
70. Cowan CL Jr, Saeed T, Stevens J, et al. Successful management of Pseudomonas endogenous endophthalmitis. Ann Ophthalmol. 1983;15:559-61.
71. Laffers Z, Bozosky S. Endogenous *Proteus* panophthalmitis. Am J Ophthalmol. 1962;54:83-8.
72. Shohet I, Davidson S, Boichis H, et al. Endogenous endophthalmitis due to *Salmonella typhimurium*. Ann Ophthalmol. 1983;15:321-2.
73. Lass JH, Varley MP, Frank KE, et al. *Actinobacillus actinomycetemcomitans* endophthalmitis with subacute endocarditis. Ann Ophthalmol. 1984;16:54-61.
74. Jampol LM, Strauch BS, Albert DM. Intraocular nocardiosis. Am J Ophthalmol. 1973;76:568-73.
75. Sher NA, Hill CW, Eifrig DE. Bilateral intraocular *Nocardia asteroides* infection. Arch Ophthalmol. 1977;95:1415-8.
76. Darrel RW. Acute tuberculous panophthalmitis. Arch Ophthalmol. 1967;78:51-4.
77. Dvorak-Theobald G. Acute tuberculous endophthalmitis. Am J Ophthalmol. 1958;45:403-7.
78. Doft BH, Kelsey SF, Wisniewski SR, the EVS Study Group. Additional procedures after the initial vitrectomy or tap-biopsy in the endophthalmitis vitrectomy study. Ophthalmology. 1998;105:707-16.
79. Maylath FR, Leopold JH. Study of experimental intraocular infection. Am J Ophthalmol. 1955;40:86-101.
80. Forster RK, Zachary IG, Cottingham AJ Jr, et al. Further observations on the diagnosis, cause, and treatment of endophthalmitis. Am J Ophthalmol. 1976;81:52-6.
81. Barza M, Pavan PR, Doft BH, et al. Evaluation of microbiological diagnostic techniques in postoperative endophthalmitis in the Endophthalmitis Vitrectomy Study. Arch Ophthalmol. 1997;115:1142-50.

82. Forster RK. Symposium: Postoperative endophthalmitis: Etiology and diagnosis of bacterial postoperative endophthalmitis. Ophthalmology. 1978;85:320-6.

83. Donahue SP, Kowalski RP, Jewar BH, et al. Vitreous cultures in suspected endophthalmitis: Biopsy or vitrectomy? Ophthalmology. 1993;100:452-5.

84. Endophthalmitis Vitrectomy Study Group. Microbiologic factors and visual outcome in the Endophthalmitis Vitrectomy Study. Am J Ophthalmol. 1996;122-830-46.

85. Brinser JH, Weiss Avery. Laboratory diagnosis in ocular disease. In: Tasman W, Jaeger EA (eds): Duane's Clinical Ophthalmology. Philadelphia, Lippincott-Raven. 1996; 4(1):1-14.

86. Joondeph BC, Flynn HW Jr, Miller D, et al. A new culture method for infectious endophthalmitis. Arch Ophthalmol. 1989;107:1334-7.

87. Isenberg SJ, Apt L, Yoshimori R, et al. Chemical preparation of the eye in ophthalmic surgery. IV. Comparison of povidone-iodine on the conjunctiva with a prophylactic antibiotic. Arch Ophthalmol. 1985;103:1340-2.

88. Apt L, Isenberg S, Yoshimori R, et al. Chemical preparation of the eye in ophthalmic surgery III. Effect of povidone-iodine on the conjunctiva. Arch Ophthalmol. 1984;102:728-9.

89. Apt L, Isenberg SJ, Yoshimori R, et al. Outpatient topical use of povidone-iodine in preparing the eye for surgery. Ophthalmology. 1989;96:289-92.

90. Speaker MG, Menikoff JA. Prophylaxis of endophthalmitis with topical povidone-iodine. Ophthalmology. 1991;98:1769-75.

91. Forster RK. Experimental postoperative endophthalmitis. Trans Am Ophthalmol Soc. 1992;90:505-59.

92. Meredith TA. Antimicrobial pharmacokinetics in endophthalmitis treatment: Studies of ceftazidime. Trans Am Ophthalmol Soc. 1993;91:653-99.

93. Stern GA. Factors affecting the efficacy of antibiotics in the treatment of experimental postoperative endophthalmitis. Trans Am Ophthalmol Soc. 1993;91:775-844.

94. May DR, Ericson ES, Peyman GA, et al. Intraocular injection of gentamicin: single injection therapy of experimental bacterial endophthalmitis. Arch Ophthalmol. 1974;91:487-9.

95. Davis JL, Koidou-Tsiligianni A, Pflugfelder SC, et al. Coagulase-negative staphylococcal endophthalmitis. Ophthalmology. 1988;95:1404-10.

96. Pflugfelder SC, Hernandez E, Fliesler SJ, et al. Intravitreal vancomycin: Retinal toxicity, clearance, and interaction with gentamicin. Arch Ophthalmol. 1987;105:831-7.

97. Conway BP, Campochiaro PA. Macular infarction after endophthalmitis treated with vitrectomy and intravitreal gentamicin. Arch Ophthalmol. 1986;104:367-71.

98. McDonald HR, Schatz H, Allen AW, et al. Retinal toxicity secondary to intraocular gentamicin injection. Ophthalmology. 1986;93:871-7.

99. Campochiaro PA, Conway BP. Aminoglycoside toxicity: A survey of retinal specialists. Arch Ophthalmol. 1991;109:946-50.

100. D'Amico DJ, Caspers-Velu L, Libert J, et al. Comparative toxicity of intravitreal aminoglycoside antibiotics. Am J Ophthalmol. 1985;100:264-75.

101. Doft BH, Barza M. Ceftazidime or amikacin: Choice of intravitreal antimicrobials in the treatment of postoperative endophthalmitis. Arch Ophthalmol. 1994;112:17-8.

102. Watanakunakorn C, Bakie C. Synergism of vancomycin-gentamicin and vancomycin-streptomycin against enterococci. Antimicrob Agents Chemother. 1973;4:120-4.

103. Watanakunakorn C, Tisone JC. Synergism between vancomycin and gentamicin or tobramycin for methicillin-susceptible and methicillin-resistant *Staphylococcus aureus* strains. Antimicrob Agents Chemother. 1982;22:903-5.

104. Campochiaro PA, Green WR. Toxicity of intravitreous ceftazidime in primate retina. Arch Ophthalmol. 1992;110:1625-9.

105. Irvine WD, Flynn HW Jr, Miller D, et al. Endophthalmitis caused by gram-negative organisms. Arch Ophthalmol. 1992;110:1450-4.

106. Lim JI, Campochiaro PA. Successful treatment of gram-negative endophthalmitis with intravitreous ceftazidime. Arch Ophthalmol. 1992;110:1686.

107. Jeglum EL, Rosenberg SB, Benson WE. Preparation of intravitreal drug doses. Ophthalmic Surg. 1981;12:355-9.

108. Bohigan GM. Intravitreal antibiotic preparation, pp.64-7. Antifungal agents. In: External diseases of the eye, Fort Worth, Alcon Laboratories. 1980.pp.158-63.

109. Paque JT, Peyman GA. Intravitreal clindamycin phosphate in the treatment of vitreous infection. Ophthalmic Surg. 1974;5:34-9.
110. Axelrod AJ, Peyman GA, Apple DJ. Toxicity of intravitreal injection of amphotericin B. Am J Ophthalmol. 1973;76:678-83.
111. Sternberg P Jr, Martin DF. Management of endophthalmitis in the post-Endophthalmitis Vitrectomy Study era. [editorial]. Arch Ophthalmol. 2001;119: 754-5.
112. The Medical Letter on Drugs and Therapeutics: The choice of antimicrobial drugs. New Rochelle, New York, Medical Letter. 1986. pp.33-40.
113. Baum J. Antibiotics use in ophthalmology In: Tasman W, Jaeger EA (eds): Duane's Clinical Ophthalmology, Philadelphia, Lippincott-Raven. 1996; 4(24):1-26.
114. O'Day DM, Foulds G, William TE, et al. Ocular uptake of fluconazole following oral administration. Arch Ophthalmol. 1990;108:1006-8.
115. Oncel M, Ercikan C. Penetration of oral fluconazole into the vitreous in humans. Invest Ophthalmol Vis Sci. 1992;33:747.
116. Jones DB. Diagnosis and management of fungal keratitis. In: Tasman W, Jaeger EA (eds): Duane's Clinical Ophthalmology. Philadelphia, Lippincott-Raven. 1996; 4(21):1-19.
117. Han DO. Corticosteroids in the management of postoperative endophthalmitis. In Syllabus: Subspecialty Day-Retina: Management of posterior segment disease, Drugs and Bugs, Dallas. 2000.pp.229-34.
118. Graham RO, Peyman GA. Intravitreal injection of dexamethasone. Treatment of experimentally induced endophthalmitis. Arch Ophthalmol. 1974;92:149-54.
119. Baum JL, Barza M, Lugar J, et al. The effect of corticosteroids in the treatment of experimental bacterial endophthalmitis. Am J Ophthalmol. 1975;80:513-5.
120. Meredith TA, Aguilar HE, Miller MJ, et al. Comparative treatment of experimental *Staphylococcus epidermidis* endophthalmitis. Arch Ophthalmol. 1990;108:857-60.
121. Maxwell DP, Brent BD, Diamond JG, et al. Effects of intravitreal dexamethasone on ocular histopathology in a rabbit model of endophthalmitis. Ophthalmology. 1991;98:1370-5.
122. Yoshizumi MO, Lee GC, Equi RA, et al. Timing of dexamethasone treatment in experimental *Staphylococcus aureus* endophthalmitis. Retina. 1998;18:130-5.

123. Liu SM, Way T, Rodrigues M, et al. Effects of intravitreal corticosteroids in the treatment of *Bacillus cereus* endophthalmitis. Arch Ophthalmol. 2000;118:803-6.

124. Mao LK, Flynn HW Jr, Miller D, et al. Endophthalmitis caused by *Staphylococcus aureus*. Am J Ophthalmol. 1993;116:584-9.

125. Das T, Jalali S, Gothwal VK, et al. Intravitreal dexamethasone in exogenous bacterial endophthalmitis: results of a prospective randomised study. Br J Ophthalmol. 1999;83:1050-5.

126. Meredith TA, Aguilar E, Drews C, et al. Intraocular dexamethasone produces a harmful effect on treatment of experimental *Staphylococcus aureus* endophthalmitis. Trans Am Ophthalmol Soc. 1996;94:241-52.

127. Kim IT, Chung KH, Koo BS. Efficacy of ciprofloxacin and dexamethasone in experimental *Pseudomonas* endophthalmitis. Korean J Ophthalmol. 1996;10:8-17.

128. Kwak HW, D'Amico DJ. Evaluation of the retinal toxicity and pharmacokinetics of dexamethasone after intravitreal injection. Arch Ophthalmol. 1992;110:259-66.

129. Smith MA, Sorenson JA, Smith C, et al. Effects of intravitreal dexamethasone on concentration of intravitreal vancomycin in experimental methicillin-resistant Staphylococcus epidermides endophthalmitis. Antimicrob Agents Chemother. 1991;35:1298-302.

130. Park SS, Vallar RV, Hong CH, et al. Intravitreal dexamethasone effect on intravitreal vancomycin elimination in endophthalmitis. Arch Ophthalmol. 1999;117:1058-62.

131. Yoshizumi MO, Bhavsar AR, Dessouki A, et al. Safety of repeated intravitreous injections of antibiotics and dexamethasone. Retina. 1999;19:437-41.

132. Hida T, Chandler D, Arena JE, et al. Experimental and clinical observations of the intraocular toxicity of commercial corticosteroid preparations. Am J Ophthalmol. 1986;101:190-5.

133. Shah GK, Stein JD, Sharma S, et al. Visual outcomes following the use of intravitreal steroids in the treatment of postoperative endophthalmitis. Ophthalmology. 2000;107:486-9.

134. Hasany SM, Basu PK, Kazden JJ. Production of corneal ulcer by opportunistic and saprophytic fungi. Can J Ophthalmol. 1973;8:119-31.

135. Coats MI, Peyman GA. Intravitreal corticosteroids in the treatment of exogenous fungal endophthalmitis. Retina. 1992;12:46-51.

136. Cottingham AJ, Forster RK. Vitrectomy in endophthalmitis: Results of study using vitrectomy, intraocular antibiotics, or a combination of both. Arch Ophthalmol. 1976;94:2078-81.

137. Talley AR, D'Amico DJ, Talamo JH, et al. The role of vitrectomy in the treatment of postoperative bacterial endophthalmitis: An experimental study. Arch Ophthalmol. 1987;105:1699-702.

138. Olson JC, Flynn HW Jr, Forster RK, et al. Results in the treatment of postoperative endophthalmitis. Ophthalmology. 1983;90:692-9.

139. Driebe WT, Mandelbaum S, Forster RK, et al. Pseudophakic endophthalmitis. Ophthalmology. 1986;93:442-8.

140. Baum J, Peyman GA, Barza M. Intravitreal administration of antibiotics in the treatment of bacterial endophthalmitis. III: Consensus. Surv Ophthalmol. 1982;26:204-6.

141. Doft BH. The Endophthalmitis Vitrectomy Study. Arch Ophthalmol. 1991;109:487-9.

142. Doft BH, Wisniewski SR, Kelsey SF, et al. Diabetes and postoperative endophthalmitis in the Endophthalmitis Vitrectomy Study. Arch Ophthalmol. 2001;119:650-6.

143. Doft BM, Kelsey SF, Wisniewski SR, for the Endophthalmitis Vitrectomy Study Group. Retinal detachment in the Endophthalmitis Vitrectomy Study. Arch Ophthalmol. 2000;118:1661-5.

144. Mao LK, Flynn HW Jr, Miller D, et al. Endophthalmitis caused by streptococcal species. Arch Ophthalmol. 1992;110:798-801.

145. Das T, Choudhury K, Sharma S, et al. Clinical profile and outcome in *Bacillus* endophthalmitis. Ophthalmology. 2001;108:1819-25.

146. Hatano H, Sasaki T, Tanaka N. Pseudomonas endophthalmitis in rabbits: intravitreal inoculation of two Pseudomonas strains. Acta Soc Ophthalmol. 1988;92:1758-64.

147. Stevens SX, Jensen HG, Jett BD, Gilmore MS. A hemolysin-encoding plasmid contributes to bacterial virulence in experimental *Enterococcus faecalis* endophthalmitis. Invest Ophthalmol Vis Sci. 1992;33:1650-6.

148. Kim IT, Park SK, Lim JH. Inflammatory response in experimental *Staphylococcus* and *Pseudomonas* endophthalmitis. Ophthalmologica. 1999;213:305-10.

149. Horio N, Terasaki H, Yamamoto E, Miyake Y. Electroretinogram in the diagnosis of endophthalmitis after intraocular lens implantation. Am J Ophthalmol. 2001;132:258-9.

11

Cystoid Macular Edema

Amar Agarwal, Priya Narang

INTRODUCTION

Since its recognition as a distinct entity by Irvine in 1953[1] and its elaborate clinical description by Gass and Norton in 1966,[2-4] aphakic and pseudophakic cystoid macular edema (CME), commonly referred to as the Irvine-Gass syndrome, has continued to perplex ophthalmologists in terms of its pathogenesis, its peculiar clinical manifestations and its treatment. It is one of the most frequent and troublesome problems following cataract surgery with or without IOL.[5-14]

MACULAR EDEMA

The extracellular space of the retina normally constitutes a small proportion of its total volume. Active transport of electrolytes and larger molecules from the retina across the retinal pigment epithelium to the blood maintains this situation. Disruption of either the inner or outer blood-retinal barrier leads to leakage of plasma proteins and water, which leads to expansion of the extracellular fluid space of the retina. This is often accompanied by accumulation of fluid in the macular area, especially in the outer plexiform layer and inner nuclear layer. Retinal edema localized to the macula is called macular edema. More generalized leakage leads to diffuse thickening of the posterior pole. Accumulation of fluid in cystic spaces leads to cystoid macular edema.

CYSTOID MACULAR EDEMA

The reason why the macula is the most commonly involved part of the retina is because of its peculiar anatomy characterized by abundance of axons (nerve fiber layer of Henle), paucity of glial tissue which holds the retinal elements together, relative lack of vasculature and greater metabolic activity.

THEORIES EXPLAINING APHAKIC AND PSEUDOPHAKIC CME

Vitreous Traction Theory

Constant constriction and dilatation of the pupil creates pulling on the anterior vitreous strands that is transmitted to the vitreous base and thence to the macula by presumed vitreous connections between the posterior hyaloid and the surface of the macula. This is the Vitreous tug syndrome.[3,15-17] Vitreoretinal adhesion is strongest at those regions where the internal limiting lamina is thinnest, i.e. the fovea and vitreous base.[18-21] In these regions, the Müller cell attachment plaques to the Internal limiting membrane are most prominent. Thus it appears that the continuity of structure between the collagen fibrils of the vitreous and the Müller cells of the retina[22] could directly transmit any movement, displacement or traction in the vitreous to the Müller cells of the macula. Since Müller cells are not only trans-retinal structural elements but also serve a vital metabolic role,[23] any damage to these cells could alter other components of the macula. Chronic Müller cell irritation may also lead to the local release of a variety of mediators, which in turn facilitates leakage.

Inflammation Theory

Eyes with CME nearly always demonstrate signs of intraocular inflammation and also respond to steroid therapy. Clinical observations associating aphakic CME with intraocular inflammation have been made for many years.[1,5,24,25] Aqueous humor contains biochemically active principles called aqueous biotoxic complex (ABC) factors,[26] which manifest biotoxic effects when it leaves its natural reservoir. If large amounts of it are produced or if there is a reduction in its absorption by the ciliary epithelium, these diffuse posteriorly through the collapsed liquefied vitreous gel. The liquefied vitreous anterior to the retina hence assumes chemical and osmotic properties quite unlike those normally present, which results in an outpouring of fluid from the perimacular capillaries. The lower incidence of CME after ECCE may be due to the presence of an intact posterior capsule that acts as a diffusion barrier.[26] The ABC factors may be prostaglandins, which are synthesized de novo. Since the eye does not contain the enzyme 15- PG dehydrogenase to deactivate prostaglandins their removal is dependant on an active transport pump called the Bito's pump located in the ciliary epithelium.[26] This pump is inoperable (overburdened or inhibited) for at least 3 weeks after ocular trauma.[27] The inflammatory state persists for longer periods when vitreous is adherent to the cataract wound causing pupillary distortion (Fig. 11.1).[28]

Anoxia Theory

This is not yet proved. An association between CME and systemic conditions, e.g. hypertension, arteriosclerotic heart disease and diabetes mellitus is seen in which anoxia could be predisposing factor for CME.[28,29]

THEORIES CONCERNING THE ORIGIN OF CYSTS OF CME

Intracellular Theory

Yanoff et al.[30] and Fine and Brucker[31] proposed that cysts develop from degenerating Muller's cells. Initially these cells demonstrate

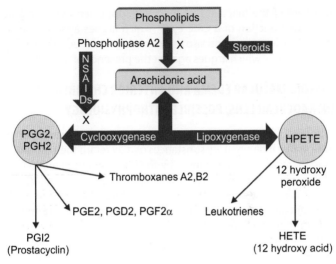

Figure 11.1 Metabolism of arachidonic acid

Abbreviations:
HPETE = Hydroperoxyeicosatetraenoic acid
HETE = Hydroxyeicosatetraenoic acid
PG = Prostaglandin
NSAIDs = Nonsteroidal anti-inflammatory drugs

edema, which gradually increases until the cytoplasm of the cells begin to develop vacuoles. The edematous cells gradually expand until the cell walls break and adjoining cells from larger cavities leading to the cysts in CME. A breakdown of the blood-retinal barrier or anoxia is the primary cause of the edema.

Extracellular Theory

Gass, Anderson and Davis[32] proposed that cysts arise from expansion of the extracellular spaces of the retina by serous exudation within the outer plexiform layer and inner nuclear layer. This involves leakage of serous exudates from perifoveal intraretinal capillaries and sometimes from disc capillaries. The exudates form small puddles in the OPL of Henle, which acts like a sponge because of the peculiar structure of the macula. This theory is supported by the highly reversible function of a CME eye,[33] which argues against cellular death and disruption, and also the visible lack of occluded capillaries in the macula, which argues against the presence of anoxia.

CYSTOID MACULAR EDEMA AND ANTERIOR CHAMBER INTRAOCULAR LENS: POSSIBLE PATHOPHYSIOLOGY

Chronic anterior uveal irritation may either stimulate production of intra ocular inflammatory substances or may retard the absorption or removal of these substances by the nonpigmented epithelium of the ciliary body. An anterior chamber intraocular lens (ACIOL), which can press against the anterior surface of the iris or apply constant pressure on the face of the ciliary body, could trigger constant anterior uveal inflammation. Older style IOL's situated with in the pupil (intracameral) that either rest upon the pupillary margin or have haptics sutured to the iris stroma possess the same, if not greater propensity to elicit chronic uveal irritation.[14] Hence, intracameral and ACIOL's are more likely to stimulate CME than are PCIOL's.[14,34,35]

INCIDENCE OF CME

Irvine[1] originally reported an incidence of 2%, but the incidence of angiographic CME is much higher, occurring approximately after 40% of intracapsular cataract extractions.[14] Also if it occurs in one eye, there is almost a 70% probability of it affecting the second eye as well after cataract surgery.[14] Phacoemulsification with "in the bag" IOL placement has been reported to have an incidence as low as 0.5%.[14] Eyes with a primary posterior capsulotomy had a significantly higher incidence of angiographic CME approximately 21.5% as compared to 5.6% in eyes with intact capsules[36,37] in one series whereas in another series no statistically significant difference was found in the incidence of angiographic CME 6 weeks or 6 months postoperatively.[38] The incidence of clinically significant pseudophakic CME after Nd: YAG laser posterior capsulotomy was around 1.23% in one study.[39]

CLINICAL APPEARANCE OF CME

Slit Lamp Examination

This is done with Hruby Lens, 90 D Lens, 78 D Lens or the Goldmann 3 mirror contact lens. Advantages are the use of slit lamp optics and stereopsis. Biomicroscopic examination with Hruby lens or a fundus contact lens or a 90 D lens shows a characteristic honey comb lesion with one or more larger cystoid spaces centrally and any number of smaller, oval spaces around them. Cystoid spaces are best seen using red free light, which makes the inner walls visible. The optical section of the convex anterior walls of the cysts can be seen overlying optically empty vesicles, tightly packed together with their interfaces presenting a spidery pattern. With the slit beam, it is possible to see a network of interlacing, fine refractile lines by retro illumination. The retina may be markedly thickened and the lesion may be as large as 1.5 to 2 disc diameters. Some cases may be associated with disc edema.

Direct Ophthalmoscopy

This usually shows a loss of foveal reflex. Monochromatic light is better for detecting subtle macular changes; hence red free light can be used. Using the macular aperture, the beam is passed slowly back and forth across the macula. The septa may be observed by retro illumination, i.e. just adjacent to the edge of the light beam. Disadvantages are the lack of stereoscopic view and the difficulty of recoding and transmitting information.

Indirect Ophthalmoscopy

This is useful in ruling out other causes of CME.

Anterior Segment Examination

This usually shows signs of inflammation. The anterior hyaloid face may be intact or broken and the vitreous usually shows cells and vitreous opacities and posterior vitreous detachment.

Fundus Fluorescein Angiography

This is used to confirm and document macular changes and for deciding the management and also for follow-up. In CME, within 1 to 2 minutes of dye injection, leakage into the macula is seen (Figs 11.2A to D). A stellate pattern with feathery margins is seen by 5 to 15 minutes usually, but sometimes taking up to 30 minutes. The pattern seen on fundus fluorescein angiography (FFA) is called the Flower Petal appearance (Fig. 11.3). The dark septae in the macular area that compartmentalize the pattern are because of the Muller's fibers. The spaces appear to intercommunicate. Usually there is considerable leakage of dye into the vitreous and aqueous anteriorly. In some patients with disc edema, there may be leakage of dye into the optic nerve and peripapillary retina.

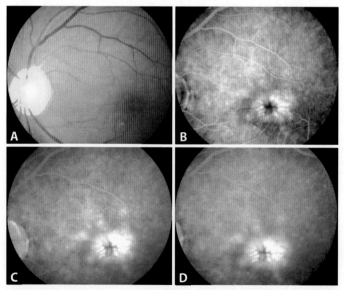

Figures 11.2 A to D A. Color fundus photograph of cystoid macular edema; Fundus fluorescein photograph of cystoid macular edema (flower petal appearance): B. Shows capillary leakage in the macular area; C. Early flower petal appearance; D. Late flower petal appearance

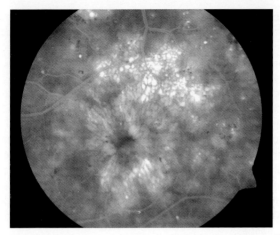

Figure 11.3 Fundus fluorescein photograph of cystoid macular edema (flower petal appearance)

Various FFA grading systems have been used for CME:[40,41]
Grade 0: No edema
Grade 1+: Capillary leakage
Grade 2+: Partial petalloid ring
Grade 3+: Complete petaloid ring

Level 1: Edema less than perifoveal
Level 2: Minimal perifoveal edema
Level 3: Moderate perifoveal edema (1 DD)
Level 4: Severe perifoveal edema

MACULAR FUNCTION TESTS IN CME

Best corrected visual acuity and visual acuity with pinhole, two-point discrimination, Maddox Rod test, and all indicate decreased macular function. Amsler grid chart may show central distortion of the grids or a relative central scotoma. The automated perimeter has special macular program, which may show central scotoma. Any blanks or scotoma in the central area on entoptic imagery implies macular involvement. Potential acuity meter (PAM) can be used for differentiating between visual loss from anterior segment disease and macular disease. Longer recovery time, up to 90 to 180 seconds on macular photostress test implies macular dysfunction even though the area may appear anatomically normal. The normal recovery time is 55 seconds. Difference between the two eyes is also significant.

In cases of opaque media, the visual acuity can be determined with clinical interferometers.

Electrophysiology[42] may also show changes in CME. Foveal electroretinogram (ERG) is a test of the temporal responsiveness of the central 10-degree of the retina and requires integrity of the outer retinal layers, especially Muller's cells. Foveal electroretinogram (FERG) is usually abnormal in 35% of CME eyes. Pattern ERG reflects the inner retinal layer function. It is usually abnormal in 53% of CME eyes. Over half of the PERG abnormal eyes had no associated FERG abnormalities.

Optical coherence tomography (OCT) should also be done in cases of CME.[43]

SEQUELA OF CME: POST-CME LAMELLAR HOLE

Permanent macular degeneration may arise secondary to prolonged chronic CME. The cystoid spaces of the macula may coalesce together so that all retinal elements disappear except for the internal limiting membrane.[14] After the internal limiting membrane also disintegrates, a lamellar hole is formed which may be one-fourth to one-third disc diameter in size.[44] Surrounding intact cystoid spaces may be seen. In the presence of a lamellar hole visual acuity may continue to be good because of the retention of some percipient elements.[26] Rarely does CME progress to a full thickness macular hole.[45,46]

ON-OFF PHENOMENON

Cystoid macular edema (CME) tends to be cyclic in nature, so that sometimes on withdrawing treatment following good response to therapy, CME may relapse again, which is called the on-off phenomenon.[41,47]

PROPHYLACTIC TREATMENT

- Steady and gentle preoperative ocular compression.
- Avoiding intracapsular cataract extraction (ICCE) and unplanned extracapsular cataract extraction (ECCE).
- Gentle tissue handling and avoiding excessive instrumentation.
- Avoiding complications like posterior capsular rent, vitreous loss, iris prolapse, etc.
- Proper management of vitreous loss with thorough anterior vitrectomy.
- In the bag IOL placement.
- IOL with chemically inert haptics and high quality optics with good surface finish and correct dimensions.
- Avoiding phototoxicity by using co-axial light only when red reflex is essential and using oblique illumination at all other times. Also by using a pupil occluder, decreasing the intensity of illumination and by rotating the macula away from light during suturing and also by using an IOL with UV absorbing optics.
- Pharmacological prophylaxis with postoperative steroids and nonsteroidal anti-inflammatory drugs (NSAIDs) through topical, subconjunctival, sub-Tenon or systemic routes. The use of steroids and NSAIDs decreases the amount of intraocular inflammatory substances released at the time of surgery.[48]

THERAPY FOR ESTABLISHED CME

Medical Therapy

- *Topical steroids:* They are given 4 to 6 times/day.
- *Repository steroid injections:* Methyl prednisolone acetate suspension (Depo-Medrol) or triamcinolone acetonide (Kenalog), usually 40 mg (1mL) is given subconjunctivally once a month. It is not to be used in eyes with a known propensity for steroid induced rise in IOP.
- *Systemic steroids:* Efficacy is not known as yet. Dosage: 40 to 100 mg/day or every alternate day.

- *Topical NSAIDs:* Topical indomethacin 1%, ketorolac 0.5% diclofenac 0.1% and flurbiprofen 0.03% can be tried. Studies have shown an improvement in vision but an on-off phenomenon[41] may be seen.
- *Oral NSAID therapy:* Indomethacin 25 mg tid after meals can be tried. Other drugs are suprofen, fenoprofen, ibuprofen, and piroxicam. All these can cause gastric irritation.
- *Hyperbaric oxygen:* Some patients receiving 2.2 atm, oxygen for 1.5 hours twice daily for 7 days and then 2 hours daily for 14 days may show improvement. Hyperbaric oxygen may help heal injured capillary complexes by causing constriction of the macular capillaries along with stimulating collagen formation that seals these spaces.[49]
- *Acetazolamide:* It facilitates transport of water across the retinal pigment epithelium (RPE) from the subretinal space to the choroid.[50] Dosage is 250 to 500 mg bid or qid.[51,52]

Medical therapy can also be tried for many elderly patients and for unwilling patients who do not want further surgery.

ND: YAG Laser Vitreolysis

This avoids an invasive procedure. Elevated vitreous strands are transected using Nd: YAG laser.[8,53] Bisecting vitreous membranes that are adherent to the anterior surface of the iris may be difficult without producing small hemorrhages which diffuse into the aqueous and make accurate focussing impossible. Therefore laser treatment is primarily used in those cases in which vitreous strands bridge the margin of the pupil to the undersurface of the cataract wound without adhering to the anterior surface of the iris.[53]

Surgical Therapy

For Aphakic CME

Vitrectomy: The goal of the surgery is to remove all formed vitreous elements from the anterior segment to restore the anatomy of the iris and pupil to a state as near normal as possible. Technique[28] – the edges of the condensed sheets of solid vitreous adherent to the anterior surface of the iris are carefully identified with the slit lamp preoperatively and with the operating microscope intraoperatively. Then a plane of dissection is created between the sheet of vitreous and the anterior surface of the iris by the to and fro swings of a micro cyclodialysis spatula introduced at 90 degree to the edge. The sheet is then removed by advancing a vitrectomy instrument beneath it. This is done till all formed vitreous is removed and the pupil is restored to normal. Next, a shallow vitrectomy is performed at the level of the pupil to prevent new strands of vitreous from finding their way to the incision site postoperatively. If a pars plana approach is used, a complete posterior vitrectomy can also be done.

For Pseudophakic CME with ACIOL

- *With relatively round pupil:* Removal of the ACIOL with anterior vitrectomy is done. The surgical aphakia is corrected either with a sulcus IOL if adequate posterior capsular rim remains (but the disadvantage here is irritation to the uveal tissue) or a scleral fixated IOL. Other solutions are contact lenses, epikeratoplasty, Excimer laser, or peripheral intrastromal corneal ring.
- *With moderate pupillary distortion from disrupted vitreous or malpositioned haptics:* Anterior vitrectomy and anterior segment restoration is done. The IOL may be left in situ or exchanged.

For Pseudophakic CME with PCIOL

- *With pupillary distortion:* Anterior segment restoration with a core pars plana vitrectomy is done.
- *With in-the-bag IOL, intact posterior capsule, normal mobile pupil, no peripheral anterior synechiae:* Here a pars plana vitrectomy could be performed to remove the vitreous sump or vitreous traction from the macula, but the sump theory is not yet proved, hence it is better not to operate. If done to release vitreo macular traction, such traction should be confirmed pre operatively by biomicroscopic examination with posterior pole contact lens.

This situation is rare and hence surgical intervention should be uncommon.[14] But before resorting to surgery in such cases, other causes for CME should be ruled out and a complete course of medical therapy should have been tried.

Key Points

- Chronic anterior uveal irritation may either stimulate production of intra-ocular inflammatory substances or may retard the absorption or removal of these substances by the nonpigmented epithelium of the ciliary body.
- Biomicroscopic examination with Hruby lens or a fundus contact lens or a 90 D lens shows a characteristic honey comb lesion with one or more larger cystoid spaces centrally and any number of smaller, oval spaces around them. Cystoid spaces are best seen using red free light, which makes the inner walls visible.
- In CME, within 1 to 2 minutes of dye injection, leakage into the macula is seen. A stellate pattern with feathery margins is seen by 5 to 15 minutes usually, but sometimes taking up to 30 minutes. The pattern seen on FFA is called the Flower Petal appearance.
- Rarely does CME progress to a full thickness macular hole.
- The goal of vitrectomy is to remove all formed vitreous elements from the anterior segment to restore the anatomy of the iris and pupil to a state as near normal as possible.

REFERENCES

1. Irvine SR. A newly defined vitreous syndrome following cataract surgery, interpreted according to recent concepts of the structure of the vitreous. Am J Ophthalmol. 1953;36:599-619.
2. Gass JDM, Norton EWD. Cystoid macular edema and papilloedema following cataract extraction: fluorescein fundoscopic and angiographic study. Arch Ophthalmol. 1966;76:646-61.
3. Tolentino FI, Schepens CL. Edema of the posterior pole after cataract extraction: A biomicroscopic study. Arch Ophthalmol. 1965;74:781-6.
4. Iliff CE. Treatment of the vitreous tug syndrome. Am J ophthalmol. 1966;62:856-9.

5. Gass JDM, Norton EWD. A follow-up study of cystoid macular edema following cataract extraction. Trans Am acad Ophthal Otolaryngol. 1969. 73:665-82.

6. Machemer R, Parel JM, Buettner H. A new concept for vitreous surgery. I Instrumentation. Am J ophthalmol. 1972;73:1-7.

7. Miyake K. Prevention of cystoid macular edema after lens extraction by topical indomethacin (I). A preliminary report. Albrecht bon graefes Arch Klin Ophthalmol. 1977;203:81-8.

8. Katzen LE, Fleischman JA,Trokel S. YAG laser treatment of cystoid macular edema. Am J Ophthalmol. 1983;95:589-92.

9. Shahidi M, Ogura Y. Correlation of retinal thickness with visual acuity in cystoid macular edema. Arch Ophthalmol. 1991;109(8):1115-9.

10. Hee MR, Puliafito CA, Wong C, et al. Quantitative assessment of macular edema with optical coherence tomography. Arch Ophthalmol. 1995;113:1019-29.

11. Arend O, Remky A, Elsner AE, et al. Quantification of cystoid changes in diabetic maculopathy. Invest Ophthalmol Vis Sci. 1995;6:608-13.

12. Wolff's Anatomy of the Eye and Orbit-Brenda and Tripathi. 8th edn. Chapman and Hall Ltd.1997.

13. Duke Elder S. System of Ophthalmology, Vol. X-Diseases of the Retina, St Louis, CV Mosby. 1967.

14. Stephen J Ryan. "Retina" 2nd edn. vol 1, 2. CV Mosby Company.

15. Jaffe NS. Vitreous traction at the posterior pole of the fundus due to alterations in the vitreous posterior. Trans Am Acad Ophthalmol Otolaryngol. 1967;71:642-52.

16. Reese AB, Jones IS, Cooper WC. Macular changes secondary to vitreous traction. Trans Am Ophthalmol Soc. 1966;64:123-34.

17. Maumenee AE. Further advances in the study of the macula, arch. Ophthalmol. 1967;78:51-165.

18. Eisner G. Biomicroscopy of the peripheral fundus. Surv Ophthalmol. 1972;17:1-28.

19. Foos RY. Vitreoretinal juncture; topographic variations. Invest Ophthalmol Vis Sci. 1972;11:801-8.

20. Grignolo A. Fibrous components of the vitreous body. Arch Ophthalmol. 1952;47:760-74.

21. Hogan MJ. The vitreous, its structure and relation to the ciliary body and retina. Invest Ophthalmol Vis Sci. 1963;2:418-45.

22. Mann I. The development of the human eye. New York, Grune and Stratton. 1964.pp.162-3.

23. Lessell S, Kuwabara T. Phosphatase histochemistry of the eye. Arch Ophthalmol. 1964;71:851-60.

24. Hitchings RA, Chisholm IH, Bird AC. Aphakic macular edema: incidence and pathogenesis. Invest Ophthalmol. 1975;14:68-71.

25. Irvine AR, Bresky R, Crowder BM, et al. Macular edema after cataract extraction. Ann Ophthalmol. 1971;3:1234-40.

26. Jaffe. Cataract surgery and its complications, 6th edition. Mosby.

27. Bito LZ, Salvador EV. Intraocular fluid dynamics. III. The site and mechanism of prostaglandin transfer across the blood intraocular fluid barriers, Exp Eye Res. 1972;14:233-41.

28. Wayne E Fung. The national, prospective, randomized vitrectomy study for chronic aphakic cystoid macular edema. Progress report and comparison between the control and nonrandomized groups, Surv Ophthalmol. 1984;28:569-75.

29. Mark OM Tso. Animal modeling of cystoid macular edema, Surv Ophthalmol. 1984;28:512-9.

30. Yanoff M, Fine BS, Brucker AJ, et al. Pathology of human cystoid macular edema. Surv Ophthalmol. 1984;28:505-11.

31. Fine BS, Brucker AJ. Macular edema and cystoid macular edema. Am J Ophthalmol. 1981;92:466-81.

32. Gass JDM, Anderson DR, Davis EB. A clinical, fluorescein angiographic, and electron microscopic correlation of cystoid macular edema. Am J Ophthalmol. 1985;100:82-6.

33. Taylor DM, Sachs SW, Stern AL. Aphakic cystoid macular edema. Longterm clinical observations. Surv Ophthalmol. 1984;28:437-41.

34. Stark WJ, Maumenee EA, Fagadau W, et al. Cystoid macular edema in pseudophakia. Surv Ophthalmol. 1984;28:442-51.

35. Moses L. Cystoid macular edema and retinal detachment following cataract surgery. J Am Intraocular Implant Soc. 1979;5:326-9.

36. Keates RH, Steinert RF, Puliafito CA, et al. Long-term follow-up of Nd:YAG laser posterior capsulotomy. J Am Intraocul Implant Soc. 1984;10:164-8.

37. Kraff MC, Sanders DR, Jampol LM, et al. Effect of primary capsulotomy with extracapsular surgery on the incidence of pseudophakic cystoid macular edema. Am J Ophthalmol. 1984;98:166-70.

38. Wright PL, Wilkinson CP, Balyeat HD, et al. Angiographic cystoid macular edema after posterior chamber lens implantation. Arch Ophthalmol.1988;106:740-4.

39. Steinert RF, Puliafito CA, Kumar SR, et al. Cystoid macular edema, retinal detachment, and glaucoma after Nd: YAG laser posterior capsulotomy. Am J Ophthalmol. 1991;112:373-80.

40. Jose' G Cunha-Vaz, Antonio Travassos. Breakdown of the blood retinal barriers and cystoid macular edema. Surv Ophthalmol. 1984;28:485-92.

41. Yannuzzi LA. A perspective on the treatment of aphakic cystoid macular edema. Surv Ophthalmol. 1984;28:540-53.

42. Salzman J, Seiple W, Carr R, Yannuzzi L. Electrophysiological assessment of aphakic cystoid macular edema. Br J Ophthalmol. 1986;70:819-24.

43. Nussenblatt RB, Kaufman SC, Palestine AG, et al. Macular thickening and visual acuity: measurement in patients with cystoid macular edema, Ophthalmology. 1987;94:1134-9.

44. Gass JDM. Lamellar macular hole: a complication of cystoid macular edema after cataract extraction—a clinic pathologic case report. Trans Am Ophthalmol Soc. 1975;73:231-50.

45. Gass JDM. Stereoscopic atlas of macular diseases: diagnosis and treatment, 3rd edn. St Louis, Mosby—Year Book, Inc. 1987.

46. Jampol LM, Sanders DR, Kraff MC. Prophylaxis and therapy of aphakic cystoid macular edema. Surv Ophthalmol. 1984;28:535-9.

47. Flach AJ, Jampol LM, Weinberg D, et al. Improvement in visual acuity in chronic aphakic and pseudophakic cystoid macular edema after treatment with topical 0.5% ketorolac tromethamine. Am J Ophthalmol. 1991;112:514-9.

48. Jampol LM. Pharmacologic therapy of aphakic and pseudophakic cystoid macular edema: 1985 update. Ophthalmology. 1985;92:807-10.

49. Ploff DS, Thorn SR. Preliminary report on the effect of hyperbaric oxygen on cystoid macular edema. J Cataract Refract Surg. 1987;13:136-40.

50. Marmor MF, Maack T. Enhancement of retinal adhesion and subretinal fluid absorption by acetazolamide. Invest Ophthalmol Vis Sci. 1982 23:121-4.

51. Cox SN, Hay E, Bird AC. Treatment of chronic macular edema with acetazolamide. Arch Ophthalmol. 1988;106;1190-5.

52. Tripathi RC, Fekrat S, Tripathi BJ, et al. A direct correlation of the resolution of pseudophakic cystoid macular edema with acetazolamide therapy. Ann Ophthalmol. 1991;23:127-9.

53. Steinert RF, Wasson PJ. Neodymium: YAG laser anterior vitreolysis for Irvine-Gass cystoid macular edema. J Cataract Refract Surg. 1989;15: 304-7.

12

Bimanual Phaco/ Phakonit/MICS: Surgical Technique

Amar Agarwal

HISTORY

On 15th August 1998, the first 1 mm cataract surgery was performed by the author (Amar Agarwal) by a technique called Phakonit.[1-3] In this the cataract was removed through a bimanual phaco technique. It was performed without any anesthesia. The first live surgery of Phakonit in the world was performed on August 22nd 1998 at Pune, India by the author (Amar Agarwal) at the Phaco and Refractive surgery conference. The major hitch with this technique was to find an IOL, which would pass through such a small incision. To overcome this a rollable IOL was introduced and on 2nd October 2001 the author (Amar Agarwal) performed Phakonit with the implantation of a rollable IOL. This was done in their Chennai (India) hospital. The lens was designed specially by Thinoptx. This lens used a Fresnel principle and was designed by Wayne Callahan from USA. The first such ultrathin lens was implanted by Jairo Hoyos from Spain. One of the authors (Am A) then modified this into a special 5 mm-optic rollable IOL.

TERMINOLOGY

The terminology PHAKONIT characterizes phaco (PHAKO) being done with a needle (N) opening via an incision (I) and with the phako tip (T). It also denotes Phako being done with a Needle Incision Technology.

SYNONYMS

- Bimanual phaco
- Micro-incision cataract surgery
- Micro-phaco
- Bimanual micro-phaco
- Sleeveless phaco.

TECHNIQUE OF PHAKONIT FOR CATARACTS

Anesthesia

The technique of Phakonit can be performed under any type of anesthesia. In the cases done by the authors no anesthetic drops were instilled in the eye nor was any intracameral anesthetic injected inside the eye. This was "no anesthesia cataract surgery".[4] The authors have analyzed that there is no difference between Topical anesthesia cataract surgery and No anesthesia cataract surgery. In complicated cases, peribulbar block is preferred.

Incision

A tuberculin syringe (1 cc) filled with viscoelastic is taken and the eye is distended by injecting viscoelastic inside the eye. The distension of the eye facilitates the creation of clear corneal incision [Note in Figure 12.1, the left hand holds a globe stabilization rod (Geuder, Germany). This helps to stabilize the eye while creating the clear corneal incision. The specially designed knife is held in the dominant hand. It creates an incision of either sub 1mm or 1.2 mm depending on which size knife is chosen by the surgeon. If the surgeon prefers

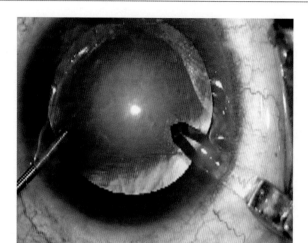

Figure 12.1 Clear corneal incision made with a special knife (MST, USA). [*Note:* The left hand has a globe stabilization rod to stabilize the eye (Geuder, Germany). This knife can create an incision from sub 1 mm to 1.2 mm]

to use a sub 1 mm knife then one should use a 21-gauge irrigating chopper and a 0.8 mm phaco needle. This keratome and other instruments for Phakonit are made by Huco (Switzerland), Gueder (Europe) and Microsurgical technology (MST, USA)].

Capsulorhexis

The capsulorhexis is then performed of approximately 5 to 6 mm in diameter. This is done with a needle (Fig. 12.2). In the left hand, a straight rod is held to stabilize the eye that is also known as the Globe stabilization rod. The advantage of this method is that the movements of the eye can be controlled as the surgeon is working without any anesthesia. Microsurgical technology (USA) has designed an excellent capsulorhexis forceps for Phakonit (Fig. 12.3) that passes through a 1 mm incision.

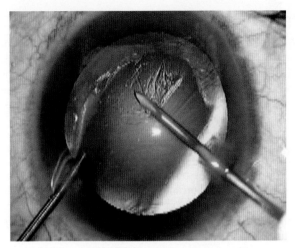

Figure 12.2 Capsulorhexis started with a needle

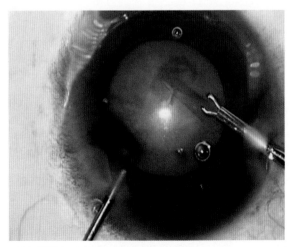

Figure 12.3 MST rhexis forceps used to perform the rhexis in a mature cataract.
(*Note:* The trypan blue staining the anterior capsule)

Hydrodissection

A 27-gauge cannula is attached to a 2 mL syringe and the cannula is introduced in to the eye. The edge of the capsulorhexis margin is lifted and a gentle fluid wave is passed beneath it. While doing so, the posterior lip of corneal incision is slightly depressed so that an outlet is available for the excess of fluid to pass out of the eye. The rotation of the nucleus is then checked.

Phakonit

After enlarging the side-port a 20 or 21 gauge irrigating chopper connected to the infusion line of the phaco machine is introduced with foot pedal on position 1. Various irrigating choppers are designed and are in use. In Figure 12.4 you will notice two designs of irrigating choppers that are designed by the author. On the left is the Agarwal irrigating chopper made by MST (Microsurgical Technology)

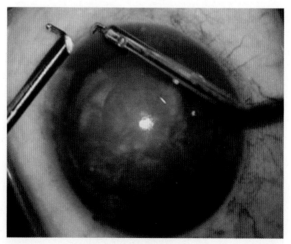

Figure 12.4 Two designs of Agarwal irrigating choppers. The one on the left has an end opening for fluid (microsurgical technology). The one on the right has two openings on the sides (Geuder, Germany)

company. This is incorporated in the Duet system (Fig. 12.5). The irrigating chopper on the right side is made by Geuder, Germany. Notice in the right the opening for the fluid is end opening, whereas the one on the left has two openings on the side. Depending on the preference of the surgeon, the surgeon can decide which design of irrigating chopper they would like to use (Fig. 12.6).

The phaco probe is connected to the aspiration line and the phaco tip without an infusion sleeve is introduced through the clear corneal incision (Figs 12.7 and 12.8). Using the phaco tip with moderate ultrasound power, the center of the nucleus is directly embedded starting from the superior edge of rhexis with the phaco probe directed obliquely downwards towards the vitreous. The settings at this stage are 50% phaco power, flow rate 24 mL/min and 110 mm Hg vacuum. When nearly half of the center of nucleus is embedded, the foot pedal is moved to position 2 as it helps to hold the nucleus due to vacuum rise. To avoid undue pressure on the posterior capsule the nucleus is lifted a bit and with the irrigating chopper in the left hand the nucleus chopped. This is done with a straight downward motion from the inner edge of the rhexis to the center of the nucleus and then to the left in the form of a laterally reversed L shape. Once the crack is created, the nucleus is split till

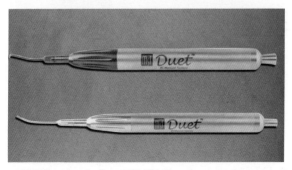

Figure 12.5 Duet handles from MST, USA. The advantage of these handles is that one can change the irrigating chopper tips

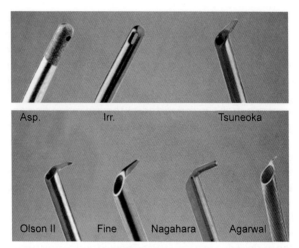

Figure 12.6 Various irrigating chopper tips designed by various surgeons. These can be fixed onto the duet handles. (MST, USA)

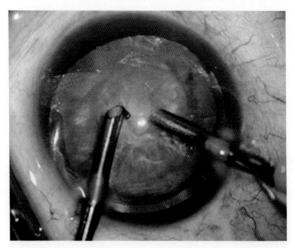

Figure 12.7 Phakonit irrigating chopper and phako probe without the sleeve inside the eye

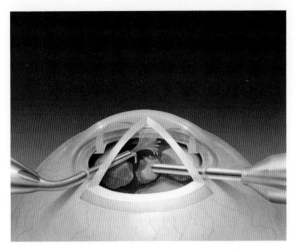

Figure 12.8 Phakonit done. Notice the irrigating chopper with an end opening. (Figure 12.12. courtesy Larry Laks, MST, USA)

the center. The nucleus is then rotated 180° and cracked again so that the nucleus is completely split into two halves.

The nucleus is then rotated 90° and embedding done in one half of the nucleus with the probe directed horizontally. With the previously described technique, 3 pie-shaped quadrants are created in one half of the nucleus. Similarly 3 pie-shaped fragments are created in the other half of the nucleus. With a short burst of energy at pulse mode, each pie shaped fragment is lifted and brought at the level of iris where it is further emulsified and aspirated sequentially in pulse mode. Thus the whole nucleus is removed. Cortical wash-up is the done with the bimanual irrigation aspiration technique (Fig. 12.9). Microsurgical Technology (USA) has also designed a soft tip irrigator-aspirator (IA) that is very safe for the posterior capsule (Fig. 12.10).

Phakonit with Cut Sleeve

During phakonit another hitch was that of splashing of the fluid from the base of the phaco needle outside the incision during

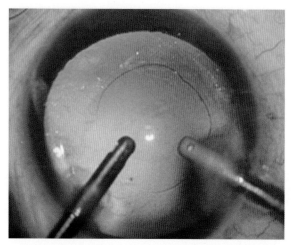

Figure 12.9 Bimanual irrigation aspiration completed

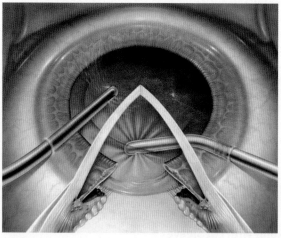

Figure 12.10 Soft tip I/A from MST, USA. (Figure 12.12. courtesy, Larry Laks, MST)

emulsification. This splashing of fluid is due to the fact that the fluid in contact with the base of the vibrating phaco needle during emulsification was churned thus releasing droplets of fluid. These fluid droplets could hamper the surgeons view directly or by getting deposited on the microscope objective.

To eliminate wound burns we should have some way of cooling the corneal wound of entry. This is usually taken care by the fluid that leaks out of the eye from the main wound as the naked phaco needle without the sleeve does not provide a water tight wound. To provide irrigation into the anterior chamber we use the irrigating chopper through the side port connected to the irrigating bottle along with an air pump specially devised for this purpose. To prevent the splashing of fluid during emulsification from the base of the phaco needle we use the cut sleeve around the base of the phaco needle. We cut the sleeve in such a manner that it covers only the base of the phaco needle and does not enter the eye. Thus we are able to prevent the splashing of fluid during emulsification.

During phakonit surgery fluid is constantly leaking out of the eye from the main wound of entry, as the incision around the phaco needle without the sleeve is not watertight. This fluid is coming from the irrigating chopper connected to the air injector. If we connect another fluid irrigating line the phaco needle with cut sleeve, fluid travels from the base of the phaco needle towards the wound of entry from outside. This stream of fluid meets the stream coming from inside eye at the corneal entry wound causing turbulence and fluid collection in the operating field. This reduces visibility during surgery. Moreover since the fluid leaking from the section cools the wound internally and the eye outwards, there is no need for the second irrigation line. More importantly when we connect the second irrigation line to the phaco hand piece with the cut sleeve, the irrigation is always on but we need it only during emulsification. Hence it is better to use an assistant who could drop cooled BSS at the external wound only during emulsification. So we advocate *"Phakonit with cut sleeve without irrigation"* to eliminate water splashing during phakonit to improve visibility during the surgery.

AIR PUMP

One of the real bugbears in Phakonit when we started it was about the problem of destabilization of the anterior chamber during surgery. This was solved to a certain extent by using an 18-gauge irrigating chopper. A development made by us (Sunita Agarwal) was to use an anti-chamber collapser [5,6] that injects air into the infusion bottle (Read Air pump chapter). This is an air pump and it pushes more fluid into the eye through the irrigating chopper and also prevents surge. Thus we had a dual benefit of using a 20-gauge irrigating chopper with no issue of destabilization of the anterior chamber during surgery. This increases the steady-state pressure of the eye making the anterior chamber deep and well maintained during the entire procedure. It even makes phacoemulsification a relatively safe procedure by reducing surge even at high vacuum levels. Thus this can be used not only in Phakonit but also in Phacoemulsification.

CRUISE CONTROL

The Cruise Control is a disposable, flow-restricting (0.3 mm internal diameter) device that is placed in between the phaco hand-piece and the aspiration tubing of any phaco machine. The goal is very similar to that of the flare tip (Alcon)—combining a standard phaco tip opening with a narrower shaft to provide more grip with less surge. David Chang and Howard Fine (USA) have popularized this for phakonit surgery. STAAR Surgical introduced this disposable Cruise Control device, which can be used with any phaco machine.

PHAKONIT CAN BE DONE WITH ANY PHACO MACHINE

The procedure of Phakonit can be done with any phaco machine currently available in the system. The parameters are:

- *Power:* 50% phaco power. Start in the continuous mode to chop the nucleus and once chopping has been done then shift to the pulse mode.

- *Suction:* 100 mm of Hg. One has to use the air pump or anti-chamber collapser so that no surge occurs. In other words some sort of forced gas infusion has to be used. One can do without it but the problem will come in difficult cases and one has to go slower.
- *Flow rate:* 20 to 24 mL/min.
- *Phaco needle:* If one uses a 0.8 mm phaco needle with a 21 gauge irrigating chopper then one can do a sub 1 mm cataract surgery. Continuous irrigation over corneal incision can be done as it negates the possibility of a corneal burn.

THINOPTX ROLLABLE IOL

Thinoptx the company that manufactures these lenses has patented technology that allows the manufacture of lenses with plus or minus 30 diopters of correction on the thickness of 100 microns. The Thinoptx technology developed by Wayne Callahan, Scott Callahan and Joe Callahan is not limited to material choice, but is achieved instead of an evolutionary optic and unprecedented nano-scale manufacturing process. The lens is made from off-the-shelf hydrophilic material, which is similar to several IOL materials already on the market. The key to the Thinoptx lens is the optic design and nano-precision manufacturing. The basic advantage of this lens is that they are Ultra-Thin lenses. One of the authors (Am A) modified this lens to make a special 5 mm optic rollable IOL.

Thinoptx have made a special injector, which not only rolls the lens but also inserts the lens. This way we do not need to use our fingers for rolling the lens. In Figure 12.11 you will notice this special injector injecting the IOL in the capsular bag. The tip of the nozzle is kept at the edge of the incision.

TOPOGRAPHY

Topography was performed with the Orbscan to compare cases of phakonit and phaco and it was concluded that the astigmatism in phakonit cases was much less compared to phaco (Fig. 12.12).

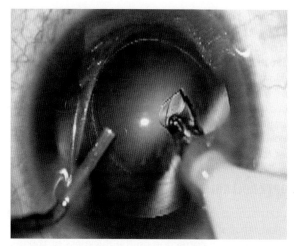

Figure 12.11 Thinoptx roller cum injector inserting the IOL in the capsular bag

Stabilization of refraction is also faster with Phakonit compared to phaco surgery. Table 12.1 compares the differences between phaco and phakonit.

ACRITEC IOL

The AcriTec company in Berlin, Germany manufactures the acrylic IOL. This lens is a sterile foldable intraocular lens made of hydrophobic acrylate. The intraocular lens consists of highly purified biocompatible hydrophobic acrylate with chemically bonded UV-absorber. It is a single piece foldable IOL like a plate-haptic IOL. The lens is sterilized by autoclaving. The lens comes in a sterile vial, filled with water and wrapped in a sterile pouch.

INTRAOPERATIVE PROTOCOL FOR VANCOMYCIN PROPHYLAXIS

Vancomycin is injected inside the eye at the end of the surgery to prevent endophthalmitis. For this the intraoperative protocol is:

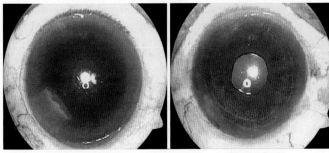

| Phacoemulsification | Phakonit with |
| with foldable IOL | Thinoptx rollable IOL |

Figure 12.12 Comparison between phaco foldable and phakonit Thinoptx IOL. The figure on the left shows a case of phaco with a foldable IOL and the figure on the right shows phakonit with a thinoptx rollable iOL

TABLE 12.1 Phaco vs phakonit		
Feature	*Phaco*	*Phakonit*
Incision size	3 mm	Sub 1.4 mm
Air pump	Not mandatory	Mandatory
Hand usage	Single handed phaco possible	Two hands (bimanual)
Non dominant hand entry and exit	Last to enter and first to exit	First to enter and last to exit
Capsulorhexis	Needle or forceps	Better with needle
IOL	Foldable IOL	Rollable IOL
Astigmatism	Two unequal incisions create astigmatism	Two equal ultrasmall incisions negate the induced astigmatism
Stability of refraction	Later than phakonit	Earlier than phaco
Iris prolapse-intraoperative	More chances	Less chances due to smaller incision

- 250 mg vial of vancomycin is taken to be dissolved in 25 mL of Ringer lactate (RL) or Balanced salt solution (BSS)
- This will give a concentration of 1 mg in 0.1 mL

- At the end of the surgery, insert 0.1 mL of vancomycin containing 1 mg into the capsular bag behind the IOL. If need be additional BSS/RL can be injected into the eye to make the eye firm.

Currently, the trend is to use intracameral moxifloxacin, which can be injected inside the eye.

CONVERSION TO PHACO OR ECCE

While performing phakonit if the surgeon experiences difficulties like corneal edema or continuous destabilization of the anterior chamber, then the surgeon should convert to phaco or extracapsular cataract extraction (ECCE).

Difficulty in doing phaco can be encountered as the side port incision is 1 mm and while doing phaco there might be fluid leakage through the side-port incision. In such a case one can suture the side port incision to make things easy. The normal chopper will be able to pass through a sutured side port and there will not be a leakage. While converting to ECCE, suturing of the clear corneal incisions should be done. The ECCE should then be performed as usual from the superior end through a scleral incision after cutting the conjunctiva.

If phakonit is continued with destabilization of the anterior chamber, permanent endothelial damage and corneal burn can be induced. Therefore, it is more prudent to convert in such cases.

SUMMARY

Hitches and glitches are a part and parcel of any new technique and so also with is the case with Phakonit. The important point is that it is now possible to do a sub-1mm incision surgery for cataract removal. This can be done comfortably by separating the phaco needle from the infusion sleeve. As the saying goes -"We have miles to go before we can sleep".

Key Points

- The technique of Phakonit can be done under any type of anesthesia. Dr Agarwal prefers the *No anesthesia cataract surgery* technique. In this no anesthetic drops are instilled in the eye nor any intracameral anesthetic is injected inside the eye. However, in difficult and challenging cases a peribulbar block is preferred.

- The capsulorhexis is preferably performed with a needle. In the left hand a straight rod is held to stabilize the eye, which is known as the globe stabilization rod. It helps to control the movements of the eye.

- Using the phaco tip with moderate ultrasound power, the center of the nucleus is directly embedded starting from the superior edge of capsulorhexis with the phaco probe directed obliquely downwards towards the vitreous. The settings kept at this stage are 50% phaco power, flow rate 24 mL/min and 110 mm Hg vacuum.

- When nearly half of the center of nucleus is embedded, the foot pedal is moved to position 2 as it helps to hold the nucleus due to vacuum rise.

- To avoid undue pressure on the posterior capsule the nucleus is lifted a bit and with the irrigating chopper in the left hand the nucleus is chopped. This is done with a straight downward motion from the inner edge of the capsulorhexis to the center of the nucleus and then to the left in the form of an inverted L shape.

- The air pump increases the steady-state pressure of the eye making the anterior chamber deep and well maintained during the entire procedure. It even makes phacoemulsification a relatively safe procedure by reducing surge even at high vacuum levels.

- The air pump should be used not only in Phakonit but also in Phacoemulsification.

- We advocate *"Phakonit with cut sleeve"* to eliminate water splashing during phakonit to improve visibility during the surgery.

- Phakonit can be done with any phaco machine available at the surgeons set up.

- The parameters in phakonit with an Alcon or AMO machine are:
  - *Power:* 50% phaco power. Start in the continuous mode and once chopping has been done then shift to the pulse mode.

Contd...

Contd...

> – *Suction:* 100 mm of Hg. One has to use the air pump or anti chamber collapser so that no surge occurs. One can do without it but the problem will come in difficult cases and one has to go slower.
> – *Flow rate:* 20 to 24 mL/min.
>
> • Vancomycin or moxifloxacin can be injected intracamerally inside the eye at the end of the surgery to prevent any occurrence of endophthalmitis.
> • During the learning curve, the surgeon can either convert to phaco or to extracapsular cataract extraction (ECCE) in case of difficulty for the best interest of the patient.

REFERENCES

1. Agarwal S, Agarwal A, Sachdev MS, Mehta K, Fine H, Agarwal A. Phacoemulsification, Laser Cataract Surgery and Foldable IOL's; 2nd edn. Jaypee Brothers Medical Publishers, New Delhi, India. 2000.
2. Boyd BF, Agarwal S, Agarwal A, Agarwal A. Lasik and Beyond Lasik; Highlights of Ophthalmology; Panama. 2000.
3. Agarwal A, Agarwal A, Agarwal S, Narang P, Narang S. Phakonit: phacoemulsification through a 0.9 mm corneal incision. J Cataract Refract Surg. 2001;27(10):1548-52.
4. Agarwal, et al. No anesthesia cataract surgery with karate chop; In: Agarwal's Phacoemulsification, Laser Cataract Surgery and Foldable IOLs, 2nd edn. Jaypee Brothers Medical Publishers, New Delhi, India. 2000. pp.217-26.
5. Fishkind WJ. The Phaco Machine: How and why it acts and reacts? In: Agarwal's Four-volume Textbook of Ophthalmology. Jaypee Brothers Medical Publishers, New Delhi, India, 2000.
6. Seibel SB. The fluidics and physics of phaco. In: Agarwal's et al. Phacoemulsification, Laser Cataract Surgery and Foldable IOLs, 2nd edn. Jaypee Brothers Medical Publishers, New Delhi, India. 2000. pp.45-54.

Microphakonit: Cataract Surgery with a 0.7 mm Tip

Amar Agarwal

HISTORY

On August 15th 1998 the author (Amar Agarwal) performed 1 mm cataract surgery by a technique called PHAKONIT.[1-13] The term 'Phakonit' means phaco being done with a needle incision technology. Dr Jorge Alio (Spain) coined the term MICS or Micro-incision cataract surgery[14] for all surgeries including laser cataract surgery and Phakonit. Dr Randall Olson (USA) first used a 0.8 mm phaco needle and a 21 gauge irrigating chopper and called it Microphaco.[15-18]

On May 21st 2005, for the first time a 0.7 mm phaco needle tip with a 0.7 mm irrigating chopper was used by the author (Am A) to remove cataracts through the smallest incision possible as of now and this was termed as 'Microphakonit'.

MICROPHAKONIT (0.7 MM) NEEDLE TIP

In my endeavor to shift to a 0.7 mm phaco needle, the point of contention was whether the needle would be able to hold the energy of the ultrasound. Larry Laks from MST, USA came up with specially designed 0.7 mm phaco needle (Fig. 13.1). The problem encountered was that with the decrease in the bore of the needle, the speed of the surgery also slows down because of the consequential decrease in the flow rate of the fluid.

It was decided to solve this problem by working on the wall of the 0.7 mm phaco needle. All phaco tips have standard wall thickness. If we consider the outer diameter to be constant, the resultant inner diameter is an area of the outer diameter minus the area of the wall. The inner diameter regulates the flow rate/ perceived efficiency (which can be good or bad, depending on how you look at it). In order to increase the allowed aspiration flow rate from what a standard 0.7 mm tip would be, it was decided to make the walls thinner, thus increasing the inner diameter. This would allow a faster surgery, which would be closer to what a 0.9 mm tip would have allowed and this would be further enhanced by gas forced infusion. Finally it was decided to go for a 30 degree tip to make it even better.

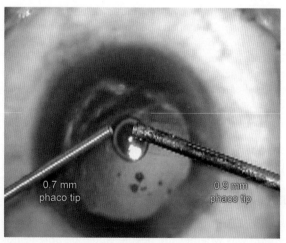

Figure 13.1 0.7 mm phaco tip (microphakonit) as compared to a 0.9 mm phaco tip (Phakonit)

MICROPHAKONIT (0.7 MM) IRRIGATING CHOPPER

There are two designs of 20 gauge (0.9 mm) irrigating choppers that we have designed. First one is the 'Agarwal irrigating chopper' made by the MST (Microsurgical Technology) company with the opening for the fluid incorporated as end openings in the Duet system. Another irrigating chopper is made by Geuder, Germany, which has two openings on the either side. Depending on the surgeon's preference, the surgeon can decide which design of irrigating chopper they would like to use. Both the choppers have their own set of advantages and disadvantages. The end opening chopper has an advantage of more fluid coming out of the chopper. The disadvantage is that there is a gush of fluid that might push the nuclear pieces away. The advantage of the side opening irrigating chopper is that there is good control as the nuclear pieces are not pushed away but the disadvantage is that the amount of fluid coming out of it is much less. It is for this reason that if one is using the side opening irrigating chopper one should use an air pump or a gas forced infusion.

The irrigating chopper made by MST helped to increase flow by removing the flow restrictions incorporated in other irrigating choppers as a by-product of their attachment method. They also had control of incisional outflow by having all the instruments to be of one size and created a matching knife of the proper size and geometry. With the incorporation of 0.7 mm irrigating chopper (Fig. 13.2), it was decided to go ahead with an end-opening irrigating chopper. The reason is as the bore of the irrigating chopper was smaller the amount of fluid coming out of it would be less and so an end-opening chopper would maintain the fluidics better. Simultaneous use of gas forced infusion helped to balance the entry and exit of fluid into the anterior chamber. The amount of fluid coming out of the various irrigating choppers with and without an air pump (Table 13.1) was calculated and properly charted out. The values using the simple aquarium air pump (external gas forced infusion) and the accurus machine giving internal gas forced infusion were also measured.

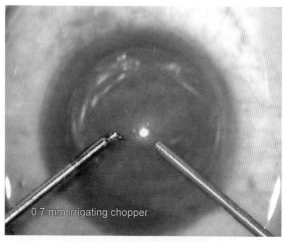

Figure 13.2 0.7 mm irrigating chopper

TABLE 13.1	Fluid exiting from various irrigating choppers (values in mL/minute)					
Irrigating chopper	Without gas forced infusion	With gas forced infusion using the accurus machine at 50 mm Hg	With gas forced infusion using the accurus machine at 75 mm Hg	With gas forced infusion using the accurus machine at 100 mm Hg	Air pump with regulator at low	Air pump with regulator at high
0.9 mm side opening	25	36	42	48	37	51
0.9 mm end opening	34	51	57	65	52	68
0.7 mm end opening	27	39	44	51	41	54

The microphakonit irrigating chopper designed by us is basically a sharp chopper that has a sharp cutting edge and helps in karate chopping or quick chopping irrespective of the density of cataract.

AIR PUMP AND GAS FORCED INFUSION

Destabilization of anterior chamber was the major problem in Phakonit surgery. Employment of an 18-gauge irrigating chopper helped to solve the problem to a certain extent. Dr Sunita Agarwal suggested the use of an antichamber collapser,[19] which injects air into the infusion bottle. This pushes more fluid into the eye through the irrigating chopper and also prevents surge (Figs 13.3 and 13.4). This ensured usage of a 20/21 gauge irrigating chopper as well as solved the problem of destabilization of the anterior chamber during surgery. Therefore with a 22 gauge (0.7 mm) irrigating chopper it is now extremely essential to use gas forced infusion in the surgery. This is also called external gas forced infusion. When the surgeon

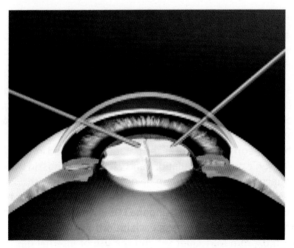

Figure 13.3 Illustration showing normal anterior chamber at the beginning of the case. Air pump is not used

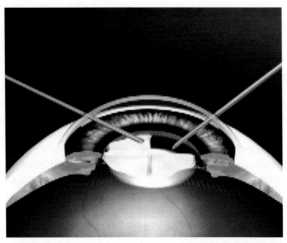

Figure 13.4 Illustration showing surge and chamber collapse when nucleus is being removed. Air pump is not used. Note the chamber depth has come down. When we use the air pump this problem does not occur

uses the air pump contained in the same phaco machine, it is called internal gas forced infusion (IFI). To solve the problem of infection, a millipore filter connected to the machine is used.

The advantages of the internal forced infusion over the external are:
- The surgeon does not have to incorporate an external air pump to the surgical system to obtain the advantages of the forced infusion.
- The surgeon can control all the parameters (forced infusion rate, ultrasonic power modulations and vacuum settings) in the same panel of the surgical system he or she is working with.
- The forced infusion rate can be actively and digitally controlled during the surgery, adjusting the parameters to the conditions and/or the surgical steps of each individual case.

With 0.7 mm MST Duet set and the use of internal gas forced infusion of the accurus machine from Alcon helped to regulate the amount of air entering into the infusion bottle and thus titrate the system in a way that there is no surge or collapse of the anterior chamber.

The anterior vented gas forced infusion system (AVGFI) of the accurus surgical system helps in the performance of phakonit. This was started by Arturo Pérez-Arteaga from Mexico. The AVGFI is a system incorporated in the accurus machine that creates a positive infusion pressure inside the eye. It consists of an air pump and a regulator that are inside the machine; then the air is pushed inside the bottle of intraocular solution, and so the fluid is actively pushed inside the eye without raising or lowering the bottle. The control of the air pump is digitally integrated in the Accurus panel. We preset the infusion pump at 100 mm Hg when we are operating microphakonit.

As depicted in Table 13.1, the use of air pump at appropriate height is equal to using the accurus machine at about 100 mm Hg pressure and if we use the air pump at low height it is equal to using the accurus machine at 50 mm Hg pressure. Some air pumps come with such a regulator so that one can have more air coming out of them. The regulator has a switch for low and high pressure and the cost of the air pump is about US $ 2 to US $ 10/- depending on the country and is available at an aquarium shop. If one uses an air pump, then it is a must to connect a millipore filter to it to prevent any infection. Alternatively one can use a gas forced internal infusion system using the accurus machine. In such a case the pump can be preset at 100 mm Hg.

BIMANUAL 0.7 MM IRRIGATION ASPIRATION SYSTEM

Bimanual irrigation aspiration is done with the bimanual irrigation aspiration cannula. These instruments are also designed by Microsurgical Technology (USA). With microphakonit the usage of specially designed 0.7 mm bimanual I/A set (Figs 13.5 and 13.6) is done so as to eliminate the need for enlarging the incision after nucleus emulsification.

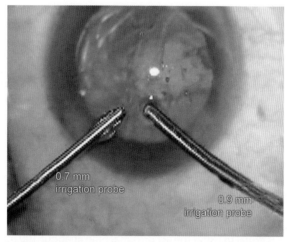

Figure 13.5 0.7 mm irrigation probe used for bimanual I/A compared to the 0.9 mm irrigation probe

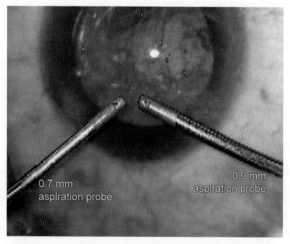

Figure 13.6 0.7 mm aspiration probe used for bimanual I/A compared to the 0.9 mm aspiration probe

DUET HANDLES

All the instruments necessary for 0.7 mm set fit onto the handles of the Duet system. So if a surgeon has already got the handles and is using it for phakonit they need to get only the tips and can use the same handles for microphakonit.

DIFFERENCES BETWEEN 0.9 MM AND 0.7 MM SETS IN CATARACT SURGERY

See Table 13.2.

TABLE 13.2 Differences between phakonit and microphakonit

Features	Phakonit	Microphakonit
Irrigating chopper	0.9 mm	0.7 mm
Phaco needle	0.9 mm	0.7 mm
Control in surgery	Good	Better control
Valve construction	Extremely important	Not very important as incision is much smaller
Iris prolapse	Can occur if valve is bad	Very rare
Intraoperative floppy iris syndrome	Can be managed	Much better to manage as incision is much smaller and there is better control
Hydrodissection	Can be done from both incisions	To be careful as very little space is there for escape of fluid
Air pump [gas forced infusion (GFI)]	Can be done without it though better with it	Mandatory 0.7 mm irrigating choppers even with higher end machines need GFI
Flow rate	Can keep any value	Do not keep it very high. 20–24 mL/min
Bimanual I/A	0.9 mm	0.7 mm

TECHNIQUE

Incision

The corneal incision is framed with a keratome, which can be either a sapphire knife or a stainless steel disposable knife. A tuberculin syringe (1cc) filled with viscoelastic is taken and viscoelastic is injected in the eye from the site where the side port has to be framed. This step helps to distend the eye before a clear corneal incision is made. It is advisable to frame one clear corneal incision between the lateral rectus and inferior rectus and the other between the lateral rectus and superior rectus. This way one is able to control the movements of the eye during surgery.

Capsulorhexis

The capsulorhexis is then performed of about 5–6 mm with a needle. In the left hand a straight rod is held to stabilize the eye with the globe stabilization rod. This helps to control the movements of the eye under 'no anesthesia' or under 'topical anesthesia'.

Hydrodissection

Hydrodissection is performed and the fluid wave passing under the nucleus is appreciated. Rotation of the nucleus is then performed. The advantage of microphakonit is that hydrodissection can be performed from both incisions so that even the subincisional areas can get easily hydrodissected. The surgeon should be careful of over hydrating or over performing the procedure as there is not much space for the fluid to escape or leak out of the eye.

Microphakonit

The 22 (0.7 mm) gauge irrigating chopper connected to the infusion line of the phaco machine is introduced with foot pedal on position 1. The phaco probe is connected to the aspiration line

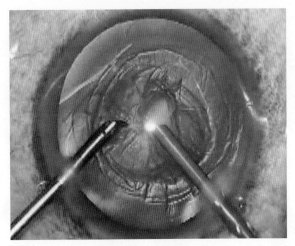

Figure 13.7 Microphakonit started. 0.7 mm irrigating chopper and 0.7 mm phako tip without the sleeve inside the eye. All instruments are made by MST, USA. The assistant continuously irrigates the phaco probe area from outside to prevent corneal burns

and the 0.7 mm phaco tip without an infusion sleeve is introduced through the clear corneal incision (Fig. 13.7). Using the phaco tip with moderate ultrasound power, the center of the nucleus is directly embedded starting from the superior edge of capsulorhexis with the phaco probe directed obliquely downwards towards the vitreous. The settings at this stage are 50% phaco power, flow rate 20 mL/min and 100–200 mm Hg vacuum. Using the karate chop technique the nucleus is chopped (Figs 13.8A to D). Thus the whole nucleus is removed (Fig. 13.9). Cortical wash-up is then done with the bimanual irrigation aspiration (0.7 mm set) technique (Figs 13.10 and 13.11). During this whole procedure of microphakonit gas forced infusion is used.

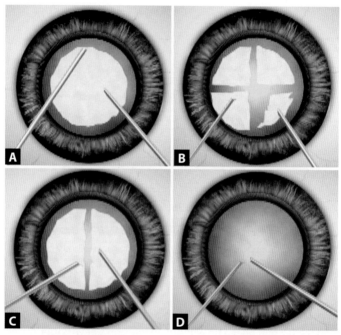

Figures 13.8A to D Illustration showing the nucleus removal

SUMMARY

With microphakonit a 0.7 mm set is used to remove the cataract. At present this is the smallest type that a surgeon one can use for cataract surgery. The problem encountered at present is the special design of an IOL needed for the procedure. There is a dearth of designing IOLs that can pass through sub 1 mm cataract surgical incisions so that the real benefit of microphakonit can be given to the patient.

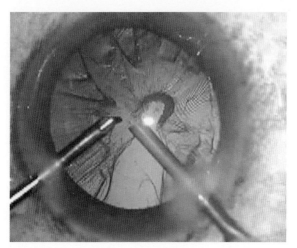

Figure 13.9 Microphakonit completed. The nucleus has been removed

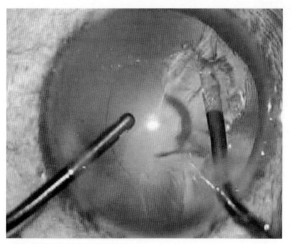

Figure 13.10 Bimanual irrigation aspiration started with the 0.7 mm set

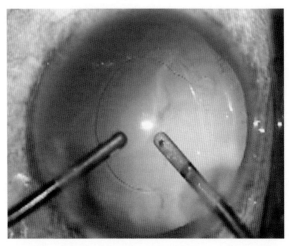

Figure 13.11 Bimanual irrigation aspiration completed

Key Points

- On May 21st 2005, for the first time a 0.7 mm phaco needle tip with a 0.7 mm irrigating chopper was used to remove cataracts through the smallest incision possible as of now. This is called Microphakonit.
- In order to increase the allowed aspiration flow rate from what a standard 0.7 mm tip would be, MST (Larry Laks) had the walls made thinner, thus increasing the inner diameter. This would allow a case to go, speed wise, closer to what a 0.9 mm tip would go (not exactly the same, but closer).
- The microphakonit irrigating chopper is basically a sharp chopper, which has a sharp cutting edge and helps in karate chopping or quick chopping. It can chop any type of cataract.
- The advantage of microphakonit is that one can do hydrodissection from both incisions so that even the sub-incisional areas can get easily hydrodissected.
- With microphakonit a 0.7 mm set is used to remove the cataract. At present this is the smallest one can use for cataract surgery. With time one would be able to go smaller with better and better instruments and devices.

REFERENCES

1. Agarwal A, Agarwal S, Agarwal At. No anesthesia cataract surgery. In: Agarwal, et al. Textbook Phacoemulsification, Laser Cataract Surgery and Foldable IOL's, 1st edn. Jaypee Brothers Medical Publishers, Delhi, India. 1998. pp.144-54.

2. Pandey S, Wener L, Agarwal A, Agarwal S, Agarwal At, Apple D. No anesthesia cataract surgery. J Cataract and Refractive Surgery. 2001; 28:1710.

3. Agarwal A, Agarwal S, Agarwal At. Phakonit: A new technique of removing cataracts through a 0.9 mm incision. In: Agarwal et al. Textbook Phacoemulsification, Laser Cataract Surgery and Foldable IOL's, 1st edn. Jaypee Brothers Medical Publishers, Delhi, India. 1998. pp. 139-43.

4. Agarwal A, Agarwal S, Agarwal At. Phakonit and laser phakonit: Lens surgery through a 0.9 mm incision. In: Agarwal, et al. Textbook Phacoemulsification, Laser Cataract Surgery and Foldable IOL's, 2nd edn. Jaypee Brothers Medical Publishers, Delhi, India. 2000. pp.204-16.

5. Agarwal A, Agarwal S, Agarwal At. Phakonit. In: Agarwal, et al. Textbook Phacoemulsification, Laser Cataract Surgery and Foldable IOL's, 3rd edn. Jaypee Brothers Medical Publishers, Delhi, India. 2003. pp.317-29.

6. Agarwal A, Agarwal S, Agarwal At. Phakonit and laser phakonit. In: Boyd/Agarwal, et al. Textbook Lasik and Beyond Lasik, Higlights of Ophthalmology, Panama. 2000. pp.463-8.

7. Agarwal A, Agarwal S, Agarwal At. Phakonit and laser phakonit—cataract surgery through a 0.9 mm incision. In: Boyd/Agarwal, et al. Textbook Phako, Phakonit and Laser Phako, Higlights of Ophthalmology, Panama. 2000. pp.327-34.

8. Agarwal A, Agarwal S, Agarwal At. The Phakonit Thinoptx IOL. In Agarwal's Textbook Presbyopia, Slack, USA. 2002. pp.187-94.

9. Agarwal A, Agarwal S, Agarwal At. Antichamber Collapser. J Cataract and Refractive Surgery. 2002;28:1085.

10. Pandey S, Wener L, Agarwal A, Agarwal S, Agarwal A, Hoyos J. Phakonit: cataract removal through a sub 1.0 mm incision with implantation of the Thinoptx rollable IOL. J Cataract and Refractive Surgery. 2002;28:1710.

11. Agarwal A, Agarwal S, Agarwal A, Narang P, Narang S. Phakonit: phacoemulsification through a 0.9 mm incision. J Cataract and Refractive Surgery. 2001;27:1548-52.

12. Agarwal A, Agarwal S, Agarwal A. Phakonit with an acritec IOL. J Cataract and Refractive Surgery. 2003;29:854-5.

13. Agarwal S, Agarwal A, Agarwal At. Phakonit with Acritec IOL. Highlights of Ophthalmology. 2000.

14. Jorge Alio: What does MICS require. In: Alios Textbook MICS; Highlights of Ophthalmology. 2004.pp.1-4.

15. Soscia W, Howard JG, Olson RJ. Micro phacoemulsification with WhiteStar. A wound-temperature study. J Cataract and Refractive Surgery. 2002;28:1044-6.

16. Soscia W, Howard JG, Olson RJ. Bimanual phacoemulsification through two stab incisions: A wound-temperature study. J Cataract and Refractive Surgery. 2002;28:1039-43.

17. Randall Olson. Microphaco chop in David Chang's textbook on Phaco Chop; Slack, USA. 2004.pp.227-37.

18. David Chang. Bimanual phaco chop in David Chang's textbook on Phaco Chop. Slack , USA. 2004.pp.239-50.

19. Agarwal A. Air pump in Agarwal's Textbook on Bimanual Phaco: Mastering the Phakonit/MICS Technique; Slack, USA. 2005.

14

Glued Intrascleral Haptic Fixation of Intraocular Lens (Glued IOL)

Amar Agarwal, Priya Narang

INTRODUCTION

Posterior capsular rent (PCR) can occur in the early learning curve in phacoemulsification.[1-15] Intraoperative dialysis or a large PCR will prevent IOL implantation in the capsular bag. Implantation of an IOL in the sulcus will be possible in cases of adequate anterior capsular support. The first glued PC IOL implantation in an eye with a deficient capsule was done on 14th Dec 2007. In eyes with inadequate anterior capsular rim and deficient posterior capsule, the new technique of IOL implantation is the fibrin glue assisted sutureless IOL implantation with scleral tuck.[3-7] Since 2007, a large number of cases have been done with this technique. The technique has also evolved since then and extended its application to many different scenarios and as part of combined surgeries. The scleral tuck and intrascleral haptic fixation of a PC IOL was first started by Gabor Scharioth from Germany.[8] Maggi had done previously a sutureless scleral fixation of a special IOL.[9]

WHITE TO WHITE MEASUREMENT

It is necessary to measure white to white (WTW) diameter and if the horizontal WTW is about 11 mm then horizontal glued IOL should be performed. This means the flaps should be made at 3 and 9 o' clock positions. If the WTW is more then it is better to do a vertical glued IOL which means the scleral flaps are made at 12 and 6 o' clock positions.

SURGICAL TECHNIQUE

Conjunctival Peritomy

If the surgeon aims at performing a manual nonphaco technique or a nonfoldable Glued IOL implantation, then it is suggested that the superior rectus muscle should be grasped and secured for better exposure. In such cases conjunctival peritomy in done in the areas where the scleral flaps are to be made. Adequate cautery should be done to stop any bleeding vessels (Fig. 14.1).

Scleral Marking

It is imperative that the scleral flaps are 180 degrees apart. If not, then the IOL will be decentered. For this reason it is better to use a scleral marker which creates marks on the cornea to see that the scleral flaps created are diagonally opposite (Fig. 14.1).

Scleral Flap Preparation

The size of the flaps should be 2.5 mm by 2.5 mm with the base at the limbus. Too large a flap is not ideal, as the haptic has to traverse a longer distance to get tucked. The surgeon should be careful so as not to make it too deep or too shallow. Once the marks are made, then a hockey flap dissector (same one which one uses to make a sclera tunnel) is taken and it is passed from one end of the flap till it comes out from the other end. The surgeon then moves the

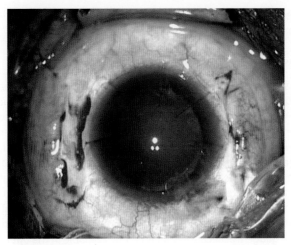

Figure 14.1 Conjunctival peritomy and scleral marking done

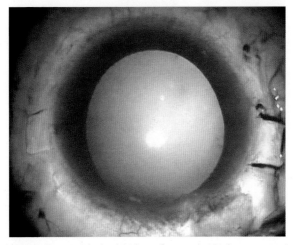

Figure 14.2 Two partial scleral thickness flaps made 180 degrees opposite to each other

dissector outwards so that the flap is created (Fig. 14.2). The flap is then lifted and any bleeding vessels can be cauterized.

Infusion with A Trocar Cannula

One should get infusion of fluid into the eye. This can be done using a sutureless 23 G/25 G trocar cannula (Fig. 14.3). The advantage is that there is no disruption of conjunctival integrity, no need for suturing the sclerotomy, and a reduction in surgical time. Insertion and removal of the cannula is faster than with a conventional 20-gauge infusion cannula. Fixating a normal 20-gauge infusion cannula requires time to cut the conjunctiva, perform cautery, and then suture the infusion cannula to the sclera. Compared with the 20-gauge infusion cannula, the 23-gauge cannula caused significantly less postoperative pain and discomfort. In summary, if a 23-gauge trocar cannula kit is readily available in the operating

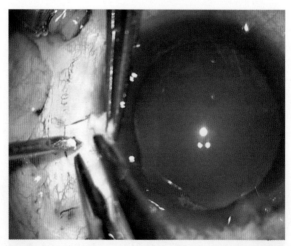

Figure 14.3 Infusion introduced into the eye with trocar-cannula. Sclerotomy being done with a 20 G needle approximately 1 mm from the limbus, beneath the scleral flaps

room, it would be easy to use in glued IOL implantation by the anterior segment surgeon.

Infusion with An Anterior Chamber (AC) Maintainer

Another alternative is to fix an AC maintainer in the eye. A clear corneal incision with a side port knife is framed and an AC maintainer is introduced into the eye. It should be kept parallel to the iris and in an area that does not affect the surgical view.

The advantage of an AC maintainer is that it is easily available and is re-autoclavable. The disadvantage is that the clear corneal incision does not always match the size of the AC maintainer accurately. This can lead to the AC maintainer coming out in the middle of the surgery and would then have to be refixed. Another issue with the AC maintainer is that when the AC maintainer fluid is turned on it pushes the iris back creating a deep anterior chamber. So when the surgeon attempts to make a 20 G needle sclerotomy under the scleral flaps, it is possible that the iris can get hit by the needle as the iris has been pushed back by the fluid from anterior chamber. This scenario can be prevented by first fixing the AC maintainer followed by creation of 20 G sclerotomies and then turning on the infusion.

Sclerotomies Under the Flap

Two straight sclerotomies with a 20 G needle are made about 1.0 mm from the limbus under the existing scleral flaps (Fig. 14.3). The sclerotomies are to be directed obliquely into the mid vitreous cavity so that the needle does not hit the iris. If 23 G Glued IOL forceps are used then 20 G sclerotomy is preferred whereas if a 22 G needle is used for sclerotomy then a 25 G Glued IOL forceps is preferred for externalizing the haptics.

Vitrectomy

Vitrectomy is performed using a 20/23/25 G vitrectomy probe (Fig. 14.4). A good vitrectomy is crucial so that there is no vitreous traction and chances of retinal breaks and retinal detachments.

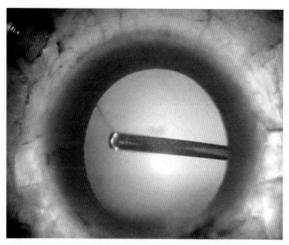

Figure 14.4 23 G vitrectomy probe introduced from the sclerotomy site. Vitrectomy being done to clear vitreous in the pupillary plane and anterior chamber

IOL Types

Glued IOL can be performed well with rigid polymethyl methacrylate (PMMA) IOL, 3-piece PC IOL, or IOLs with modified PMMA haptics. Therefore, an entire inventory of special sutured scleral fixated SFIOLs with eyelets is not needed. In dislocated PC PMMA IOL or 3-piece IOLs, the same IOL can be repositioned thereby reducing the need for further manipulation. It is safest to use a 3-piece foldable IOL as the haptics do not break as compared to a single piece non-foldable IOL. The length of a normal foldable 3-piece IOL that is available in India is 13 mm.

Foldable IOL Injectors

It is preferable to have a plunger-type injector for better coordination although a screwing mechanism type injector may also be used. In the latter case, the assistant gently maneuvers the IOL forward as the surgeon holds the injector with one hand and the glued IOL forceps with the other hand. While introducing the injector, it is advisable to have the injector tip within the mouth of the incision and not use wound-assisted injection of the IOL that can lead to a sudden, uncontrolled entry of the IOL into the eye and a consequent IOL drop into the vitreous.

Leading Haptic Externalization

Once the lens is loaded, the haptic is slightly protruded out of the cartridge and it is then introduced into the AC. The glued IOL forceps is passed through the sclerotomy and it grasps the tip of the haptic (Fig. 14.5). The IOL is then gradually injected into the eye. Once the optic has totally unfolded inside the eye, the tip of the leading haptic is pulled and is externalized (Fig. 14.6). The haptic is then grasped by an assistant (Fig. 14.7).

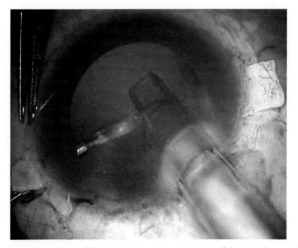

Figure 14.5 A 3-piece foldable IOL loaded and being unfolded in the eye. The tip of the leading haptic is grasped with MST forceps (Glued IOL forceps)

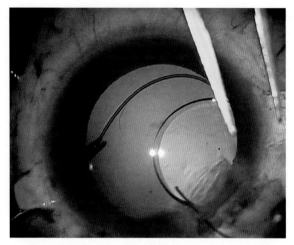

Figure 14.6 The surgeon waits for the entire IOL to unfold

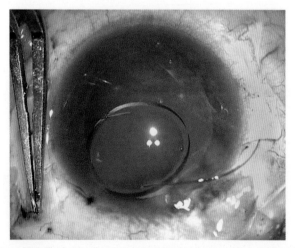

Figure 14.7 The leading haptic is externalized and grasped by an assistant to prevent its slippage into the eye

Trailing Haptic Externalization

The trailing haptic is caught with the glued IOL forceps and flexed into the AC (Fig. 14.8). The haptic is transferred from the first forceps to the second using the handshake technique. The second forceps is passed through the side port. The first forceps is then passed through the sclerotomy under the scleral flap. The haptic is transferred from the second forceps back to the first using the hand shake technique once again (Fig. 14.9). The haptic tip is grasped with the first forceps and pulled towards the sclerotomy and externalized.

Vitrectomy Around the Sclerotomy

While all these maneuvers are being done some vitreous might be present in the sclerotomy site. Vitrectomy should be done around the sclerotomy (Fig. 14.10) site to cut down all the protruding vitreous strands.

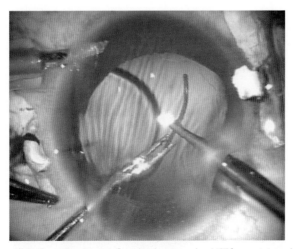

Figure 14.8 The trailing haptic is flexed in the eye and an MST forceps is introduced from the side port incision. The trailing haptic is then grasped by left hand

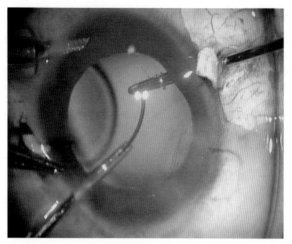

Figure 14.9 The surgeon withdraws the right hand and re-introduces the MST forceps from the right sclerotomy site. The haptic is then transferred from left to right hand

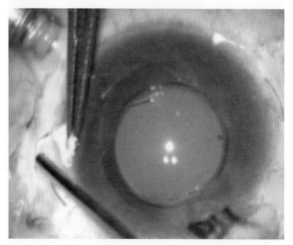

Figure 14.10 Vitrectomy done at sclerotomy site to cut down all vitreous strands

Scharioth Scleral Pocket and Intrascleral Haptic Tuck

Gabor Scharioth from Germany started the first intrascleral haptic fixation in 2006. It is the intrascleral haptic fixation which gives stability to the IOL. A 26 G needle is taken and a scleral tunnel is made at the edge of the flap where the haptic is externalized. The haptic is then flexed and tucked into the scleral pocket (Figs 14.11 to 14.13). One can also mark the Scharioth scleral pocket and create it even before the eye is opened. The 26 G needle is marked with the marker pen to leave a mark in the sclera where the scleral pocket is created. This can be done adjacent to the area where the sclerotomy will be made. This facilitates localization of the opening of the pocket due to its staining with the dye.

Air in the AC

Air is now injected into the AC and the fluid from the infusion cannula is turned off. Injection of air in the AC allows to have a firm globe intra- and postoperatively (Fig. 14.14).

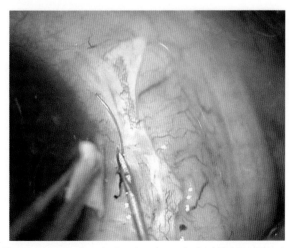

Figure 14.11 Site for scleral pocket chosen. It should be parallel to the sclerotomy site and along the edge of the scleral flap wall

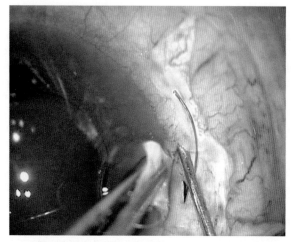

Figure 14.12 Scleral pocket made with a 26 G needle

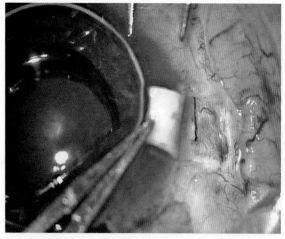

Figure 14.13 Haptic tucked in scleral pocket

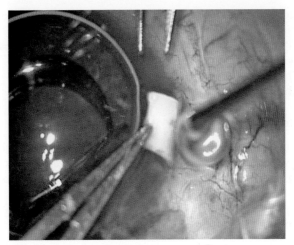

Figure 14.14 Fibrin glue applied beneath the scleral flaps for adhesion

Fibrin Glue

The fibrinogen and thrombin are first reconstituted according to the manufacturer's instructions. The commercially available FG is virus inactivated and is checked for viral antigen and antibodies with polymerase chain reaction; hence, the chances of transmission of infection are very low. The glue is applied beneath the flaps (Fig. 14.14) and after sealing them it can be used over the conjunctiva and clear corneal incisions to seal them too.

Role of Fibrin Glue

The fibrin glue plays a multifactorial role in Glued IOL surgery.
- The glue helps seal the haptic to the sclera which gives extra support to the intrascleral haptic tuck
- The glue seals the flaps so that there is no opening from inside the eye to the outside. This prevents any chances of endophthalmitis even some years later where one could get conjunctivitis leading

to endophthalmitis as there is an opening from inside to the outside of the eye
- The glue prevents any trabeculectomy opening as the flaps are now firmly stuck
- The glue helps seal the cut conjunctiva
- The glue helps seal the clear corneal incisions.

Postoperative Regimen

It comprises of topical antibiotic and steroid drops at frequent intervals throughout the day for the first postoperative week. The drugs are then tapered sequentially over a follow-up period of 2 months.

Stability of the IOL Haptic

As the flaps are manually created, the rough apposing surfaces of the flap and bed heal rapidly and firmly around the haptic, being helped by the fibrin glue early on. The major uncertainty here is the stability of the fibrin matrix in vivo. Numerous animal studies have shown that the fibrin glue is still present at 4–6 weeks. Because postoperative fibrosis starts early, the flaps become stuck secondary to fibrosis even prior to full degradation of the glue. The ensuing fibrosis acts as a firm scaffold around the haptic which prevents movement along the long axis (Fig. 14.15). To further make the IOL rock stable, we tuck the haptic tip into the scleral wall through a tunnel. This prevents all movement of the haptic along the transverse axis as well (Fig. 14.16). The stability of the lens first comes through the tucking of the haptics in the scleral pocket created. The tissue glue then gives it extra-stability and also seals the flap down. Externalization of the greater part of the haptics along its curvature stabilizes the axial positioning of the IOL and thereby prevents any IOL tilt.

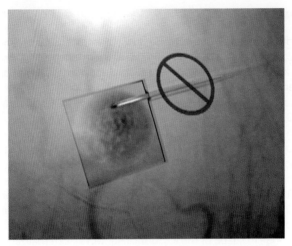

Figure 14.15 Any longitudinal movement of the haptic is avoided due to tucking

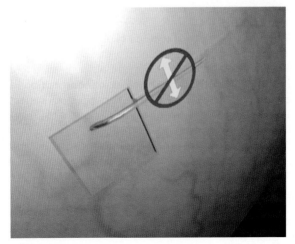

Figure 14.16 Horizontal movement of the haptic is nullified by tucking

ADVANTAGES

This fibrin glue assisted sutureless PC IOL implantation technique would be useful in a myriad of clinical situations where scleral fixated IOLs are indicated, such as, luxated IOL, dislocated IOL, zonulopathy or secondary IOL implantation.

- *No special IOLs needed*: It can be performed well with rigid PMMA IOL, 3 piece PC IOL or IOLs with modified PMMA haptics. One therefore, does not need not to have an entire inventory of special SFIOLs with eyelets, unlike in sutured SFIOLs. In dislocated posterior chamber PMMA IOL, the same IOL can be repositioned thereby reducing the need for further manipulation.

- *No tilt*: Since the overall diameter of the routine IOL is about 12 to 13 mm, with the haptic being placed in its normal curved configuration and without any traction, there is no distortion or change in shape of the IOL optic (Fig. 14.17). Externalization of the greater part of the haptics along its curvature stabilizes the axial positioning of the IOL and thereby prevents any IOL tilt.

- *Less pseudophacodonesis*: When the eye moves, it acquires kinetic energy from its muscles and attachments and the energy is dissipated to the internal fluids as it stops. Thus pseudophacodonesis is the result of oscillations of the fluids in the anterior and posterior segment of the eye. These oscillations, initiated by movement of the eye, result in shearing forces on the corneal endothelium as well as vitreous motion lead to permanent damage. Since the IOL haptic is stuck beneath the flap, it would prevent the further movement of the haptic and thereby reducing the pseudophacodonesis.

- *Less UGH syndrome*: We expect less incidence of UGH syndrome in fibrin glue assisted IOL implantation as compared to sutured scleral fixated IOL. This is because; in the former the IOL is well stabilized and stuck onto the scleral bed and thereby, has decreased intraocular mobility whereas in the latter, there is increased possibility of IOL movement or persistent rub over the ciliary body.

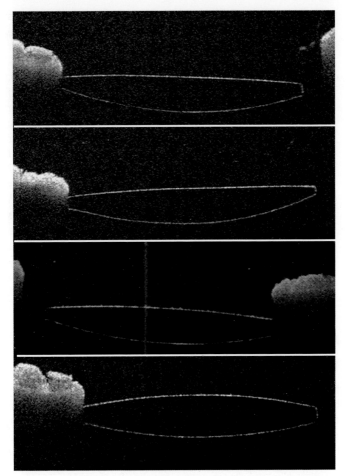

Figure 14.17 Optical coherence tomography (OCT) shows no optic tilt

- *No suture related complications*: Visually significant complications due to late subluxation that has been known to occur in sutured scleral fixated IOL may also be prevented as sutures are totally avoided in this technique. Another important advantage of this technique is the prevention of suture related complications like suture erosion, suture knot exposure or dislocation of IOL after suture disintegration or broken suture.

- *Rapidity and ease of surgery*: Since all the time taken in SFIOL for passing suture into the IOL haptic eyelets, to ensure good centration before tying down the knots as well as time for suturing scleral flaps and closing conjunctiva are significantly reduced. The risk of retinal photic injury which is known to occur in SFIOL would also be reduced in our technique due to the short surgical time. Fibrin glue takes less time [Reliseal (20 seconds)/Tissel (3secs)] to act in the scleral bed and it helps in adhesion as well as hemostasis. The preparation time can also be reduced in elective procedures by preparing it prior to surgery as it remains stable up to 4 hours from the time of reconstitution. Fibrin glue has been shown to provide airtight closure and by the time the fibrin starts degrading, surgical adhesions would have already occurred in the scleral bed. This is well shown in the follow up anterior segment OCT (Fig. 14.18) where postoperative perfect scleral flap adhesion is observed.

MODIFICATIONS IN GLUED IOL SURGERY

Three Hands in Glued IOL Surgery

Normally in a glued IOL surgery, the assistant holds the leading haptic while the surgeon engages in the externalization of the trailing haptic. A definite part of surgical expertise is required for the assistant to hold the haptic properly. Undue pressure on the haptic causes it to flatten which is then difficult to tuck. Inability of the assistant to hold the leading haptic along the correct plane causes IOL torsion while externalization and renders the procedure difficult at times.

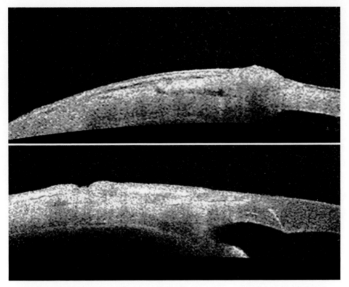

Figure 14.18 Well adhered scleral flaps seen on anterior segment OCT

No Assistant Technique (NAT)

'No Assistant Technique'[16, 17] is an effort to decrease the dependence on the assistant and make it more surgeon dependent. This technique is an attempt to make the process of 'externalization of haptics' that is considered to be the most technically demanding part of the surgery; more easy and feasible. The concept of no assistant technique was conceptualized by one of us (PN).

Physics: The entire technique works on the simple principle of physics. The vector forces. The mid-pupillary plane is the major contributor to the success of this technique.

Normal Scenario: After externalization of the leading haptic, there is a tendency of the haptic to slip back into the anterior chamber due to vector forces acting along the axis of the IOL. Green arrow indicates the vector forces.

No Assistant Technique: When the trailing haptic crosses the mid-pupillary plane and is nearly at 6 o'clock position, the vector forces act in a way that causes further extrusion of the leading haptic from the sclerotomy site with virtually no chance of slippage of leading haptic into the anterior chamber.

Needle-guided Intrascleral Fixation of Posterior Chamber Intraocular Lens for Aphakia Correction

Iñaki Rodríguez-Agirretxe and others from, Instituto Clínico Quirúrgico de Oftalmología, Vizcaya, Spain came out with this concept. A 3-piece IOL is inserted into the anterior chamber and the IOL is then rotated so the tip of the haptic to be externalized faces the scleral flap. Using a 25-gauge needle, a straight sclerotomy is made 1.0 mm from the sclera-corneal limbus. The haptic is guided into the needle and the needle withdrawn. This ensures that the haptic is also withdrawn with the needle. Then intrascleral haptic fixation can be done.

Beiko and Steinert's Modification

Dr Roger Steinert and Dr George Beiko[18] suggested the use of silicon tires or plugs to prevent slippage of leading haptic into the eye. The technique of Glued IOL requires an assistant to hold the haptics of the IOL once they have been externalized through the sclerotomies. If an assistant is not available, it is likely that the externalized haptic will be pulled into the eye once the second haptic is externalized. In order to prevent the migration of the first haptic into the eye, it is possible to use a silicone tire or a plug. The silicone tires are readily available from a Mackool Capsular Support System (Impex Surgical) or MST Capsular Support (Microsurgical Technology Inc.). Placing the silicone tire on the haptic provides support for the haptic while the entire procedure is performed.

Toshihiko Ohta's Y-fixation Technique

Toshihiko Ohta from Japan started a simplified and safer method of sutureless intrascleral posterior chamber intraocular lens fixation. This is called the Y-Fixation technique.

Key Points

- Glued IOL allows safe and secure implantation of a secondary IOL.
- A 3-piece foldable IOL is the preferred choice for implantation in a glued IOL surgery.
- Although a 1-piece IOL can also be implanted, it requires lot of surgical expertise to perform, as there are chances of breaking the haptic during the process of externalization.
- Vitrectomy should be performed at the sclerotomy site to prevent vitreous traction in future.
- Before applying fibrin glue beneath the flaps, infusion should be turned off to prevent the eventual washout of the glue by the fluid. The scleral bed should be properly dried up before its application.
- Various modifications of glued IOL surgery have propped up which offer more independence to the surgeon and eliminate the need of an assistant.

REFERENCES

1. Vajpayee RB, Sharma N, Dada T, et al. Management of posterior capsule tears. Surv Ophthal. 2001;45:473-88.
2. Wu MC, Bhandari A. Managing the broken capsule. Curr Opin Ophthalmol. 2008;19:36-40.
3. Agarwal A, Kumar DA, Jacob S, et al. Fibrin glue–assisted sutureless posterior chamber intraocular lens implantation in eyes with deficient posterior capsules. J Cataract Refract Surg. 2008;34:1433-8.
4. Prakash G, Kumar DA, Jacob S, et al. Anterior segment optical coherence tomography–aided diagnosis and primary posterior chamber intraocular lens implantation with fibrin glue in traumatic phacocele with scleral perforation. J Cataract Refract Surg. 2009;35:782-4.
5. Prakash G, Jacob S, Kumar DA, et al. Femtosecond assisted keratoplasty with fibrin glue–assisted sutureless posterior chamber

lens implantation: a new triple procedure. J Cataract Refract Surg. In press (manuscript no 08-919).

6. Agarwal A, Kumar DA, Prakash G, et al. Fibrin glue–assisted sutureless posterior chamber intraocular lens implantation in eyes with deficient posterior capsules [Reply to letter]. J Cataract Refract Surg. 2009; 35:795-6.

7. Nair V, Kumar DA, Prakash G, et al. Bilateral spontaneous in-the-bag anterior subluxation of PC IOL managed with glued IOL technique: A case report, Eye Contact Lens 2009. In Press (manuscript no ECL-07-281).

8. Gabor SGB, Pavilidis MM. Sutureless intrascleral posterior chamber intraocular lens fixation. J Cataract Refract Surg. 2007;33:1851-4.

9. Maggi R, Maggi C. Sutureless scleral fixation of intraocular lenses. J Cataract Refract Surg. 1997;23:1289-94.

10. Teichmann KD, Teichmann IAM. The torque and tilt gamble. J Cataract Refract Surg. 1997;23:413-8.

11. Jacobi KW, Jagger WS. Physical forces involved in pseudophacodonesis and iridodonesis. Albrecht Von Graefes Arch Klin Exp Ophthalmol.1981;216:49-53.

12. Price MO, Price FW Jr, Werner L, et al. Late dislocation of scleral-sutured posterior chamber intraocular lenses. J Cataract Refract Surg. 2005;31(7):1320-6

13. Solomon K, Gussler JR, Gussler C, Van Meter WS. Incidence and management of complications of transsclerally sutured posterior chamber lenses. J Cataract Refract Surg. 1993;19:488-93.

14. Asadi R, Kheirkhah A. Long-term results of scleral fixation of posterior chamber intraocular lenses in children ophthalmology. 2008;115(1):67-72. Epub 2007 May 3.

15. Lanzetta P, Menchini U, Virgili G, et al. Scleral fixated intraocular lenses: an angiographic study. Retina. 1998;18:515-20.

16. Narang P. Modified method of haptic externalization of posterior chamber intraocular lens in fibrin glue–assisted intrascleral fixation: No-assistant technique. J Cataract Refract Surg. 2013;39:4-7.

17. Narang P. Postoperative analysis of glued intrascleral fixation of intraocular lens and comparison of intraoperative parameters and visual outcome with 2 methods of haptic externalization. J Cataract Refract Surg. 2013;39:1118-9.

18. Beiko G, Steinert R. Modification of externalized haptic support of glued intraocular lens technique. J Cataract Refract Surg. 2013;39:323-9.

15

Glued IOL with Add on Procedures

Priya Narang, Amar Agarwal

GLUED IOL SCAFFOLD

Introduction

The first glued posterior chamber intraocular lens (IOL) implantation in an eye with a deficient capsule was done on 14th Dec 2007. Since 2007, a large number of cases have been done with this technique.[1-6] In 2011, we started a technique to prevent nuclear fragments from falling into the vitreous cavity called the IOL scaffold technique.[7] We hereby describe a technique that combines the glued IOL with the IOL scaffold thus creating an artificial posterior capsule in cases of posterior capsular rupture (PCR).

Concept and Indications

In the IOL Scaffold technique we implant a three piece foldable IOL above the iris or over the anterior capsule in cases of PCR. This prevents the nuclear pieces from descending into the vitreous, as the IOL acts as a scaffold or a temporary platform. Once the nucleus is emulsified the same IOL can then be placed into the sulcus or glued to the sclera depending on the availability of the anterior capsule.

The problem comes in cases in which the iris support is not sufficient and if with that there is no anterior capsular support to support the IOL scaffold technique. In such cases we cannot implant the IOL to support the nuclear pieces as then the IOL may sink. This can happen in cases like an iris coloboma (Fig. 15.1) in which a PCR has occurred and there is no capsular support at all. Alternatively in cases like a floppy iris where the iris is not taught enough to support the IOL or cases in which the pupil is very dilated and not constricting due to trauma and once again there is no capsular support.

Surgical Technique

In cases of intraoperative PCR, the phacoemulsification procedure is withheld. The remaining nuclear pieces are brought into the anterior chamber. An infusion cannula is fixed and scleral flaps are fashioned as in glued IOL surgery (Figs 15.2 and 15.3). Sclerotomy is then created with a 20-gauge needle approximately 1 mm behind the limbus under the scleral flaps. A 23 G vitrectomy probe is passed through the sclerotomy to perform vitrectomy so that all the tractional forces in the vitreous are nullified. Vitrectomy is an essential step in the surgery as one can otherwise land up with a retinal detachment postoperatively.

The three-piece foldable IOL is loaded onto the injector and the cartridge passed into the anterior chamber (AC). The haptic tip should be slightly out of the cartridge so that when one goes to grasp the haptic with the glued IOL forceps it is easy. The haptic tip is grasped with the glued IOL forceps and while the IOL is unfolded the haptic tip is still caught. The chances of the IOL falling down are not there as the haptic is caught with the forceps and the trailing haptic is still outside the clear corneal incision. Using the handshake technique the trailing haptic is externalized. If the nuclear pieces are occupying a lot of space in the AC this maneuver is sometimes difficult. One should use viscoelastic to dislodge the pieces to the side to gain visualization.

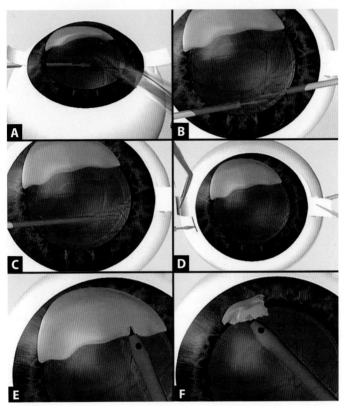

Figures 15.1A to F Glued IOL Scaffold Illustrative steps: A. Intraoperative posterior capsular rupture (PCR) noted. Nuclear pieces brought to the anterior chamber. Preparation for glued IOL surgery. Scleral flaps created. Three piece foldable IOL implantation. Note the cartridge in the AC. Also note the haptic is slightly out of the cartridge so that it is easy for the glued IOL forceps to grasp the tip of the haptic; B. Handshake technique; C. Handshake technique completed; D. Both haptics externalized; E. Phaco of the nuclear pieces. Artificial posterior capsule created by the IOL; F. Nucleus emulsified. Note the IOL Scaffold and the Glued IOL procedure combined prevent the nucleus from falling down. Nucleus totally emulsified

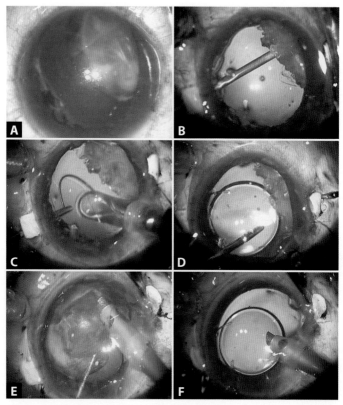

Figures 15.2A to F Glued IOL Scaffold for subluxated traumatic cataract: A. Traumatic subluxated cataract; B. Vitrectomy; C. Three piece foldable IOL implantation. Note the cartridge in the AC; D. Both haptics externalized; E. Phaco of the nuclear pieces. Artificial posterior capsule created by the IOL; F. Nucleus emulsified. Note the IOL Scaffold and the glued IOL procedure combined prevent the nucleus from falling down. Nucleus totally emulsified

A 26 G needle is used to create the Scharioth pocket and the haptics are tucked into the intrascleral pocket. Phacoemulsification of the nuclear pieces is then performed as an artificial posterior

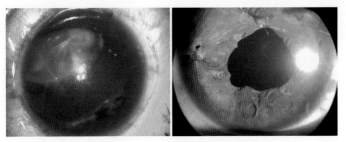

Figure 15.3 Pre and post after glued IOL scaffold

capsule has been created using the combination of the glued IOL and the IOL scaffold technique. This prevents the nuclear fragments from falling into the vitreous cavity. Finally air is injected into the AC and fibrin glue is used to seal the scleral flaps.

Difficulties

The biggest problem encountered during the procedure is the visualization of haptics in cases of large nuclear fragments. Another precaution to follow is to be careful of endothelial damage as phacoemulsification procedure is performed in the anterior chamber. Profuse use of viscoelastic is advocated to prevent endothelial damage.

Combining the glued IOL and the IOL scaffold techniques, the surgeon can create an artificial posterior capsule in certain select cases of capsular deficiency where the iris is deficient or the pupil is too large to support an IOL.

PRE-DESCEMET'S ENDOTHELIAL KERATOPLASTY WITH GLUED IOL

Surgical Considerations for Combined Procedure

The main advantage of combining Pre-Descemet's endothelial keratoplasty (PDEK) and glued IOL surgery is patient convenience.

Patients undergo only one surgery, attend fewer appointments, and deal with only one set of postoperative medications.

Although a combined surgical procedure is not significantly more complex than PDEK surgery alone, a few concerns must be addressed, especially for novice surgeons. During the surgery, the surgeon must be prepared for a decreased view secondary to guttata or haze, decreased anterior chamber stability (in cases requiring explantation of a previous IOL), increased chances of graft dislocation (intraoperative miosis is often required), increased intraocular inflammation that may lead to increased endothelial cell damage, and a potential risk of problems with the anterior chamber air fill due to air diversion into the vitreous.

Surgical Technique

The initial step involves successful harvesting of the donor lenticule followed by Glued IOL procedure (minus the application of glue to seal the scleral flaps) followed by recipient bed preparation and donor lenticule insertion. Application of fibrin glue to seal the scleral flaps is then ensued so as to ensure that it is not washed off by the fluids emanating and egressing from the eye.

Step 1: Donor graft preparation (Figs 15.4A to D).

The detailed method of preparation of donor graft has been previously described.[8] To mention in brief, an air filled 5 mL syringe with an attached 30 G needle is introduced from the corneoscleral disc with bevel up till the center of the donor lenticule with the endothelial side up. As air is injected, a Type 1 bubble is formed with a distinct edge all around. A trephine of suitable diameter is used to create a mark on the endothelium. The edge of the bubble at extreme periphery is perforated followed by injection of trypan blue into the bubble to stain the graft, which is then cut all around the trephine mark with corneoscleral scissors. The graft is then stored in the storage media.

Step 2: In cases of previously existing AC IOL, the scleral tunnel is fashioned and the AC IOL is removed from the eye. If the case has a

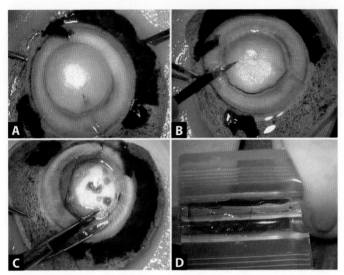

Figures 15.4A to D Donor graft preparation in pre-Descemet's endothelial keratoplasty (PDEK): A. With the endothelial side up, a 30 G needle attached to a 5 mL syringe is introduced from the periphery and air is injected so as to create a Type-1 bubble that characteristically spreads from center to periphery; B. The edge of the big bubble (bb) is penetrated with a side-port blade; C. Trypan blue is injected inside the bubble so as to stain the graft. The graft is then cut along its peripheral edge and is harvested; D. The graft is loaded on to the injector of a foldable IOL

PC IOL in the AC the same IOL is glued into the posterior chamber. Glued IOL technique[9] consists of making two partial scleral thickness flaps approximately 2.5 by 2.5 mm in size and 180 degrees opposite to each other (Figs 15.5 to 15.7). The epithelium of the recipient eye is often debrided due to epithelium decompensation, which hinders the intraoperative view to a great extent. An anterior chamber (AC) maintainer is introduced in the lower quadrant and a sclerotomy wound is created with a 20 G needle approximately 1 mm away from limbus beneath the scleral flaps and the entire glued IOL surgery is performed till the tucking of the haptics in the scleral pockets.[10] AC maintainer helps to maintain the AC through out the surgery and the use of viscoelastic is deterred as it is important not to leave residual viscoelastic in the anterior chamber as it is thought to potentially hamper good adhesion between the donor corneal disc and the recipient corneal stroma.

Step 3: The recipient cornea is marked with a trephine so as to outline the area of DM to be excised. A reverse sinskey hook is introduced into the anterior chamber and descematorhexis is performed corresponding to the margins of the epithelial mark. The DM is then stripped off and is removed from the anterior chamber. The donor pre-Descemet's roll is loaded on to the cartridge of a foldable IOL injector and the spring of the injector is removed (as originally improvised by Francis Price) so as to prevent any damage to the donor graft. The donor roll is injected into the anterior chamber and the graft is slowly unfolded with air and fluidics avoiding any direct contact with the graft so as to minimize the trauma. The PDEK graft rolls like a DMEK graft with the endothelium on the outer side, although due to the splinting effect of PDL the rolling of tissue graft is comparatively less. After proper orientation of the graft, air is injected beneath it to facilitate proper adhesion to the posterior corneal stroma. About 30 minutes is allowed to elapse to facilitate initial donor recipient corneal disc adherence. Fibrin glue is then applied beneath the scleral flaps and the incisions are sealed. Postoperatively, the patient is asked to lay flat in the recovery room for about an hour and also to lay flat for the most part during the first postoperative day.

After surgery, all patients undergo pressure patching and supine positioning overnight. Beginning the next morning, 0.1% dexamethasone sodium phosphate and moxifloxacin eye drops are administered every 2 hourly for 1 week and the every 4 hourly for next 3 weeks. Topical steroid drops are then tapered to 3 times daily in the second month, twice daily in the third month, and once daily from the fourth month onward.

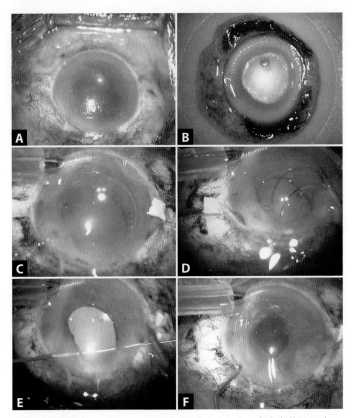

Figures 15.5A to F It takes two to tango- Pre-Descemet's endothelial keratoplasty (PDEK) with glued IOL: A. Preoperative photograph of the cornea of the patient with pseudophakic bullous keratopathy. PC IOL in AC; B. A type-1 big bubble (bb) between the pre-Descemet's layer (Dua's layer) and stroma is formed. Note the bb does not reach the periphery of the cornea as there are firm adhesions between the pre-Descemet's layer and stroma in the periphery. If a bubble is created that extends to the corneoscleral limbus it is a type-2 (pre-Descemet's) bb that symbolizes that the air has formed between the Descemet's membrane and the Pre-Descemet's layer; C. AC maintainer is fixed and sclera flaps created; D. Glued IOL surgery is performed and haptics are externalized; E. Pupilloplasty; F. Pupilloplasty completed with glued IOL in place. Eye is now ready for PDEK surgery

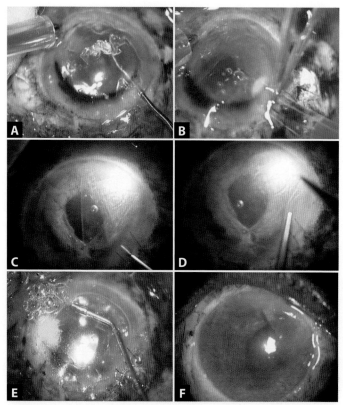

Figures 15.6A to F It takes two to tango- Pre-Descemet's endothelial keratoplasty with glued IOL: A. Descematorhexis being performed; B. The PDEK graft is injected into the anterior chamber with the help of the injector; C. Graft is subsequently unrolled with air and fluidics. An endo-illuminator is used to help in ascertaining orientation and checking the unrolling of the graft (E-PDEK); D. The graft is unrolled after checking correct orientation; E. Air is injected under the graft to appose it to the cornea. PDEK graft is attached to the cornea with a complete air fill of the anterior chamber. Then glue applied to the scleral flaps; F. Postoperative one week image of the patient

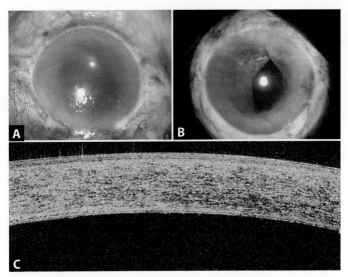

Figures 15.7A to C It takes two to tango- Pre-Descemet's endothelial keratoplasty with glued IOL: A. Preoperative case of pseudophakic bullous keratopathy with a PC IOL placed in the AC; B. Postoperative one month 20/30 vision after PDEK and glued IOL; C. Anterior segment OCT showing the graft attached

Refractive Concern

Performing IOL implantation before a corneal procedure involves lot of refractive instability and unpredictable keratometry values; therefore, predicting the lens implant power before a corneal procedure can present challenges. Studies of lens power calculations associated with keratoplasty have shown that an effective way of reducing postoperative ametropia is to perform keratoplasty first, followed by lens extraction and IOL implantation at a later date. Flowers et al. reported 95% of patients within ±2.00 D of intended postoperative target refraction following PKP and cataract extraction with IOL placement performed secondarily.

REFERENCES

1. Agarwal A, Kumar DA, Jacob S, et al. Fibrin glue–assisted sutureless posterior chamber intraocular lens implantation in eyes with deficient posterior capsules. J Cataract Refract Surg. 2008;34:1433-8.

2. Prakash G, Kumar DA, Jacob S, et al. Anterior segment optical coherence tomography–aided diagnosis and primary posterior chamber intraocular lens implantation with fibrin glue in traumatic phacocele with scleral perforation. J Cataract Refract Surg. 2009;35:782-4.

3. Prakash G, Jacob S, Kumar DA, et al. Femtosecond assisted keratoplasty with fibrin glue–assisted sutureless posterior chamber lens implantation: a new triple procedure. J Cataract Refract Surg. In press (manuscript no 08-919).

4. Agarwal A, Kumar DA, Prakash G, et al. Fibrin glue–assisted sutureless posterior chamber intraocular lens implantation in eyes with deficient posterior capsules [Reply to letter]. J Cataract Refract Surg. 2009;35:795-6.

5. Nair V, Kumar DA, Prakash G, et al. Bilateral spontaneous in-the-bag anterior subluxation of PC IOL managed with glued IOL technique: A case report, Eye Contact Lens 2009. In Press (manuscript no ECL-07-281).

6. Gabor SGB, Pavilidis MM. Sutureless intrascleral posterior chamber intraocular lens fixation. J Cataract Refract Surg. 2007;33:1851-4.

7. Kumar DA, Agarwal A, et al. IOL Scaffold technique for posterior capsular rupture. J Refract Surg. 2012;28(5):314-5.

8. Agarwal A, Dua HS, Narang P, et al. Pre-Descemet's endothelial keratoplasty (PDEK). Br J Ophthalmol. 2014(9) 1181-5. doi:10.1136/bjophthalmol. 2013;304639.

9. Dua HS, Faraj LA, Said DG, et al. A novel pre-Descemet's layer (Dua's layer). Ophthalmology. 2013;120:1778-85.

10. Agarwal A, Kumar DA, Jacob S, et al. Fibrin glue-assisted sutureless posterior chamber intraocular lens implantation in eyes with deficient posterior capsules. J Cataract Refract Surg. 2008;34:1433-8.

IOL Scaffold

Amar Agarwal, Priya Narang

INTRODUCTION

A breach in the continuity of the posterior capsule is a cause of concern. Posterior capsular rupture (PCR) is a dreaded complication of cataract surgery; it jeopardizes the chances of inserting a posterior lens and therefore obtaining the ideal optical correction. The purpose of modern cataract surgery is to maintain the integrity of the posterior capsule, not only to support the intraocular lens (IOL), but to diminish the incidence of retinal complications like cystoid macular edema and retinal detachment.

The PCR develops most frequently during removal of the last nuclear fragment following a transient postocclusion surge, especially when dealing with a dense nucleus.[1] Early recognition and proper management of PCR are important as they limit the size of the capsule tear, minimize vitreous loss, and avert the disaster of a dropped nucleus. The conventional management consists of prevention of mixture of cortical matter with vitreous, dry aspiration, and anterior vitrectomy. In addition, during phacoemulsification low flow rate, high vacuum, and low ultrasound are advocated if a posterior capsule tear occurs.

The IOL scaffold procedure[2,3] is intended for use in cases where PCR occurs with a nonemulsified, moderate to soft nucleus. A three-piece foldable IOL acts as a scaffold or a barrier to compartmentalize the anterior and posterior chambers, thereby preventing the vitreous prolapse, vitreous hydration and nucleus drop.

SURGICAL TECHNIQUE

The surgery is performed under peribulbar anesthesia. Upon recognition of a PCR, dispersive viscoelastic is injected to seal the capsular break from the side port incision without withdrawal of the phaco probe. After adequate sealing of the rent, the phaco probe is withdrawn and dispersive OVD is used to levitate and bring all the nuclear remnants into the anterior chamber (Fig. 16.1A). In cases of small PCR's, the tear is converted into a posterior capsulorhexis; whereas in cases of large tears it is difficult to do so. A 23/25 G vitrectomy probe is introduced with high cutting rate and adequate suction parameters. The infusion needle can be used to maintain the anterior chamber during vitrectomy; care being taken so that the fluid does not push the nuclear fragments down. The direction of the flow should be beneath the nuclear fragment towards the pupillary area. The pupillary area is cleared of vitreous and the presence of any strand is confirmed with the use of triamcinolone acetonide 0.5 cc injection. A 3-piece foldable IOL is injected beneath the nuclear fragment in a way that the leading haptic is guided and placed above the capsulorhexis while the trailing haptic is left extruded at the corneal incision (Figs 16.1B and C; Figs 16.3A and B). The phacoemulsification probe is introduced into the eye and the nuclear fragments are emulsified (Figs 16.1D, 16.2A, 16.3C and D). Using a dialer in the nondominant hand, the surgeon maneuvers the optic-haptic junction on the trailing haptic side so that the IOL blocks the pupil (Fig. 16.2B). Keeping the trailing haptic outside the incision enables adjustment of the IOL position in case if the nucleus rotates thus reducing the risk of IOL drop. Any residual cortex is then removed using the vitrectomy probe in suction mode with

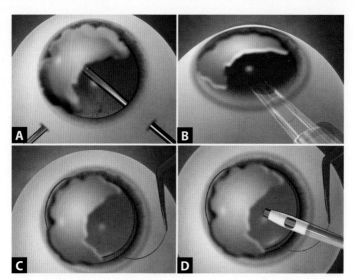

Figures 16.1A to D Animated demonstration of IOL scaffold: A. Nuclear remnants are lifted in to the anterior chamber; B. A 3-piece foldable intraocular lens (IOL) being injected beneath the nuclear remnant; C. Trailing haptic left extruded from the corneal incision; D. Phacoemulsification probe being introduced above the IOL

low aspiration. The IOL is maneuvered over the capsular remnants in the ciliary sulcus (Figs 16.2C and D, 16.3E and F). If the capsular support is inadequate, a glued IOL procedure is performed. The infusion cannula/anterior chamber maintainer is removed, and the trailing haptic is then dialed into position above the capsulorhexis and the stability of the IOL checked. The incisions are hydrated and checked for stability.

DISCUSSION

Posterior capsular rupture is a known complication of cataract surgery. The incidence of this complication is higher amongst trainees but it can occur in the hands of experienced surgeon's

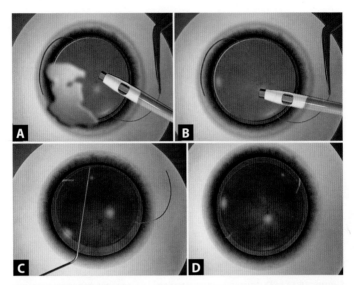

Figures 16.2A to D Animated demonstration of IOL scaffold: A. Nuclear remnants being emulsified; B. Phacoemulsification complete; C. IOL being dialed in to sulcus; D. Well placed IOL above capsulorhexis

too.[4,5] Loss of vitreous cause's significant ocular morbidity and its appropriate management is an important aspect of cataract surgery.[6]

After the posterior capsule rupture, removal of residual lens material is a challenging but important goal. Sequential, interdependent strategies to accomplish this include the Viscoat PAL, the Viscoat Trap, bimanual pars plana anterior vitrectomy, and bimanual irrigation–aspiration of cortex. Once brought into the anterior chamber, the nucleus can be removed either with phacoemulsification above a Sheet's glide, or by converting to a manual extracapsular cataract extraction approach.[7]

The dispersive viscoelastic serves as an effective barrier to vitreous prolapse while preventing posterior dislocation of lens

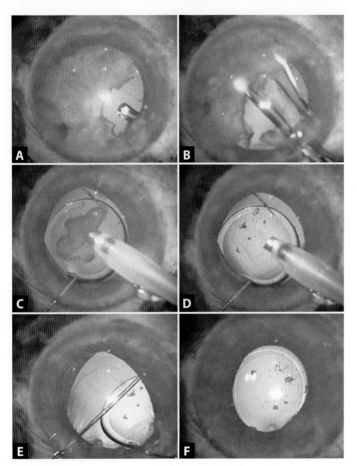

Figures 16.3A to F Clinical pictures of IOL scaffold technique: A. Vitrectomy being done beneath the nuclear fragments; B. A 3- piece foldable injected beneath the nuclear remnants; C. Phacoemulsification being done. The IOL acts as a scaffold and prevents the drop of nuclear material in the vitreous cavity; D. Phacoemulsification complete; E. IOL being dialed in to sulcus; F. IOL in sulcus

material. Viscodissection or manually moving the remaining lens material up out of the remaining capsule and into the anterior chamber can be done from where it can be safely emulsified and aspirated.[8,9] A pars plana sclerotomy to inject the supplemental supporting viscoelastic behind the nucleus, and then using the cannula tip to elevate the nuclear fragments forward through the pupil, under direct microscopic visualization.

The IOL scaffold is a technique aimed at preventing complications and achieving a successful visual outcome after posterior capsular rupture. As the IOL is inserted through the existing corneal incision, this technique has an advantage of maintaining anterior chamber stability and the intraocular pressure (IOP) while preserving the astigmatic benefits of sutureless, small incision surgery.

As the name suggests, a three-piece IOL acts as a temporary platform or a scaffold, preventing nuclear fragments from falling into the vitreous cavity.

The technique can be used after the nuclear fragments are brought into the anterior chamber, but it should be limited to the management of PCR in eyes with soft to moderate nuclei, considering the risk of corneal damage in cases of hard cataract. The advantages with this technique are that it establishes a physical barrier to nucleus drop without any need to enlarge the phacoemulsification incision. Also there is no need for sutures that might induce postoperative astigmatism. Preventing nucleus fragments from falling into the vitreous eliminates added risks from secondary surgery for large dropped fragment removal. In conclusion, IOL Scaffold can be done successfully with low complication rates with the aid of 3-piece IOL serving as a scaffold for the nuclear remnants in patients with posterior capsular rupture.

IOL SCAFFOLD FOR IOL EXCHANGE

The IOL scaffold to facilitate IOL exchange[10] is a technique that has been done in collaboration with Dr Roger Steinert and Dr Brian Little. They have significantly contributed to its development and have successfully employed it in their patients with postcataract refractive surprize.

Unpredictable refractive error following a cataract surgery can be a major cause of dissatisfaction to the patient. In such a scenario, intraocular lens (IOL) exchange for the correction of refractive surprize becomes imperative. Improper IOL power calculation, incorrectly labeled IOL's, intraoperative error by surgeon in placing the IOL at a different position as desired preoperatively during the IOL power calculation or an error on the part of an assistant while delivering the IOL to the surgeon during surgery can account for some of the potential reasons leading to an IOL exchange.

IOL scaffold is a technique described for facilitating emulsification of the nuclear fragments in cases with inadvertent posterior capsule rupture wherein the IOL is preplaced beneath the nuclear fragments thereby acting as a scaffold. In cases of IOL exchange, after levitating the offending IOL from the capsular bag, the corrective IOL can be preplaced in the bag before the offending IOL is cut and explanted out of the eye. In this way, the corrective IOL acts as a scaffold when the offending IOL is cut and it also prevents any inadvertent damage to the posterior capsule during the procedure of bisection of the offending IOL. The IOL power is re-calculated by using formulas, which have been described in the literature. Availability of the case sheet of the patient, which denotes the IOL power of the previously implanted IOL in the eye, can be of great help and it can facilitate in determining the corrective power after taking residual refractive error into consideration.

A corneal tunnel incision is framed and viscoelastic is injected in to the eye (Fig. 16.4) so as to coat the endothelium adequately. In long standing cases, adhesions between the margin of the anterior capsule and the optic of the IOL can be encountered. These adhesions can be broken down after passing a rod like structure or an iris spatula beneath the anterior capsule margin. Once the adhesions are freed, adequate amount of viscoelastic is injected beneath the optic of the IOL so as to create a space between the posterior capsule and the posterior surface of the IOL. The edge of

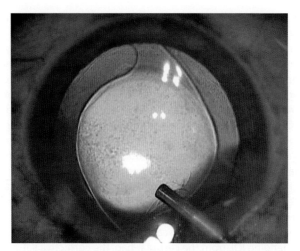

Figure 16.4 Viscoelastic being injected inside the eye

the optic is lifted with Y-shaped rod (Fig. 16.5) and the offending IOL is slowly manipulated out of the capsular bag (Fig. 16.6). The foldable corrective IOL is loaded on to the cartridge and is slowly injected beneath the offending IOL so as to place it in the capsular bag (Fig. 16.7). The corrective IOL is then dialed in to position. With an IOL cutting scissor, the offending IOL is cut along its longitudinal axis, across the optic (Fig. 16.8). The IOL is then rotated 180 degrees and is again cut along the precut axis so as to divide it in to two pieces (Fig. 16.9). The edge of the haptic is then grasped and the cut hemi-section of the IOL is pulled out of the eye followed by removal of the residual hemi-section too (Figs 16.10 and 16.11). Bimanual irrigation aspiration is then performed and the viscoelastic is removed from the eye. Stromal hydration is done and a 10-0 nylon suture is taken to seal the corneal section if need arises.

This procedure serves as an effective tool to facilitate the explantation of an IOL. In eyes with shallow anterior chamber or less anterior chamber depth, adequate attention should be imparted to the endothelium due to the proximity of the offending IOL to

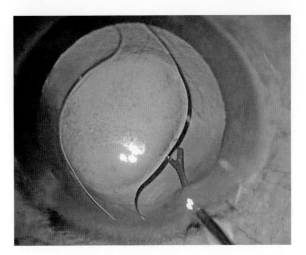

Figure 16.5 The edge of the optic is lifted with a rod

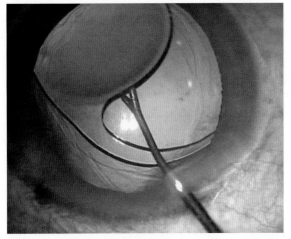

Figure 16.6 The offending IOL being manipulated out of the capsular bag

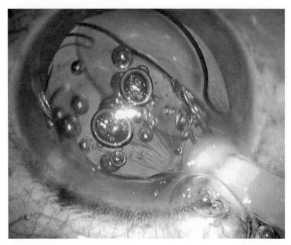

Figure 16.7 The offending IOL lying in anterior chamber and the corrective IOL is being injected in to the capsular bag

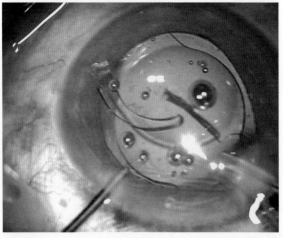

Figure 16.8 The offending IOL is cut across its optic, along the longitudinal axis

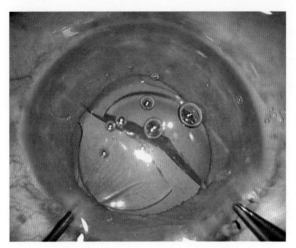

Figure 16.9 The offending IOL is rotated and the optic is bisected

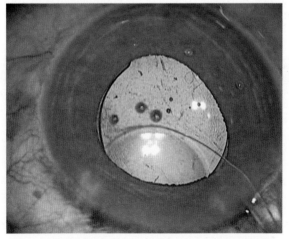

Figure 16.10 The bisected IOL is pulled by its haptic and is explanted

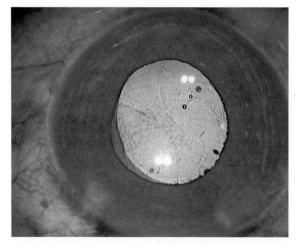

Figure 16.11 The offending IOL is completely removed from the anterior chamber. The corrective IOL is safely placed in the bag

the cornea. Adequate coating of the endothelium with dispersive viscoelastic is recommended in such cases.

Key Points

- IOL scaffold is a procedure that compartmentalizes the eye in a case of PCR and facilitates the emulsification of the residual nuclear material.
- A 3-piece foldable IOL is inserted below the nuclear fragments that acts as a scaffold.
- Another application of IOL scaffold procedure is for an IOL exchange. The offending IOL is levitated in to the anterior chamber from the bag. The corrective IOL is then injected beneath the offending IOL and is then dialed in to the bag. The offending IOL is then cut with an IOL cutting scissors and is explanted out of the eye. During the process of cutting the IOL, the corrective IOL acts as a scaffold for the posterior capsule and prevents any inadvertent cutting or damage to the posterior capsule.

REFERENCES

1. Soon-Phaik Chee. Pseudo anterior capsule barrier for the management of posterior capsule rupture. J Cataract Refract Surg. 2012;38:1309-15.
2. Kumar DA, Agarwal A, Prakash G, et al. IOL scaffold technique for posterior capsular rupture. J Refract Surg. 2012;28:314-5.
3. Narang P, Agarwal A, Kumar DA, et al. Clinical outcomes of intraocular scaffold lens surgery. A one year study. Ophthalmology. 2013;120(12):2442-8.
4. A Haripriya, D Chang, Mascarenhas Reena, M Shekhar. Complication rates of phacoemulsification and manual small-incision cataract surgery at Aravind Eye Hospital. J Cataract Refract Surg. 2012;38:1360-9.
5. Unal M, Yucel I, Sarıcı A, Artunay O, Devranoglu K, Akar Y, et al. Phacoemulsification with topical anesthesia: resident experience. J Cataract Refract Surg. 2006;32:1361-5.
6. Reddy MK. Complications of cataract surgery. Indian J Ophthalmol. 1995;43:201-9.
7. Posterior Capsular Rupture During Cataract Surgery. Laura J Ronge Eye Net Magazine 200509.
8. Michela Cimberle B. Four strategies help manage posterior capsule rupture with nucleus present Viscoat PAL, the Viscoat "trap," bimanual pars plana vitrectomy and bimanual I&A can prevent dropped lens material. OSN Europe Asia Edition, October 2002.
9. Agarwal A, "IOL scaffold," presented at Refractive Surgery Subspecialty Day session "Lull Before the Storm. A Video-Based Session" at the annual meeting of the International Society of Refractive Surgery, Orlando, Florida, USA, October 2011.http://www.aao.org/isrs/resources/outlook/11/11_11_feat.cfm. Accessed March 1, 2012.
10. Narang P, Steinert R, Little B, Agarwal A. Intraocular lens scaffold to facilitate intraocular lens exchange. J Cataract Refract Surg. 2014;40 (9):1403-7.

17

Pars Plicata Anterior Vitrectomy

Amar Agarwal, Priya Narang

INTRODUCTION

Posterior capsule rupture (PCR) while the nucleus is yet to be emulsified is a precipitous and intimidating complication that puts the surgeon on a high 'adrenaline rush'. A PCR is always an unwelcomed situation and is a cataract surgeon's nightmare. This complication is often further precipitated by the constriction of pupil and inability to do a proper vitrectomy as desired by the surgeon.

A limbal incision vitrectomy (Fig. 17.1), which is a preferred site by most of the anterior segment surgeons, often leads to the collapse of anterior chamber and an improper access to the lenticular matter trapped in the pupillary plane. Potential limitations of this approach include the fixed directionality of the instruments and cannula, which may lead to corneal distortion and poor visualization, and the fulcrum effect of the cannula may restrict the instrument movement too.

Pars plana (Fig. 17.2) has always been a favored choice of sclerotomy site for vitrectomy and retinal surgeries due to various reasons. In literature, limbal based and pars plana vitrectomy are the two well defined methods of performing a thorough vitrectomy following a PCR. The idea to choose pars plicata as a route for

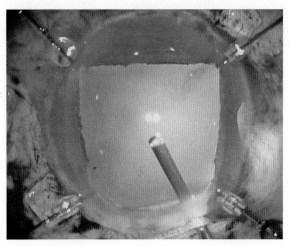

Figure 17.1 Limbal incision vitrectomy. (*Note:* The scleral incision through which vitrectomy is being done)

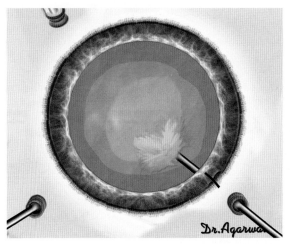

Figure 17.2 Pars plana vitrectomy

performing a thorough anterior vitrectomy crept in from the technique of glued IOL surgery; where a sclerotomy is made at the level of pars plicata (Figs 17.3 and 17.4) followed by vitrectomy from

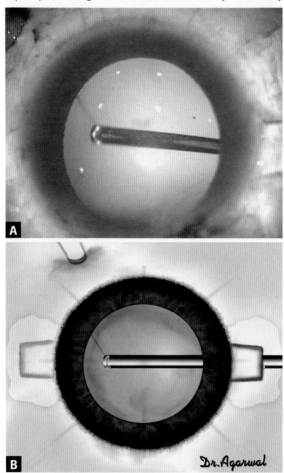

Figures 17.3A and B Pars plicata vitrectomy: A. Operative image; B. Illustrative image

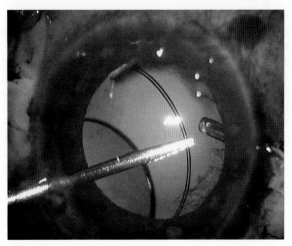

Figure 17.4 Pars placta vitrectomy for glued IOL surgery in a subluxated IOL case. (*Note:* The glued IOL forceps (Epsilon, USA) holding the haptic of the IOI to prevent it from falling down)

the same site. Invariably, pars plicata site is an underutilized option for performing anterior vitrectomy. Anterior segment surgeons always fear to tread this path as the sclerotomy site is 3.5 mm away from the limbus and is very close to the vitreous base and peripheral retina. Surgical complications related to the insertion and removal of instruments through the pars plana incisions during vitrectomy has been well described. Retinal breaks and dialyses posterior to the sclerotomy are known to occur intraoperatively owing to the mechanical traction on anterior vitreous.

SURGICAL TECHNIQUE

Following a PCR, adequate amount of viscoelastic is injected in the eye from the side port incision before the withdrawal of the phaco probe. The main corneal incision is sutured with 10-0 nylon and an anterior chamber maintainer is introduced into the eye. Minimal conjunctival peritomy is done around the site from where MVR blade is to be introduced. With a vernier caliper, around 1.5 mm away from the limbus, a 20 gauge MVR blade is introduced in an obliquely downward direction. A 23 gauge vitrectomy probe is introduced from this site and a thorough vitrectomy is done to debulk the vitreous in the pupillary plane. The anteriorly prolapsed vitreous is addressed through the posterior capsule tear. Precautions are taken to avoid extending the capsule tear and protecting the anterior capsulorhexis margin. The capsular bag and residual capsule support are assessed to determine the final placement of an IOL. In cases of good sulcus support, a 3-piece foldable IOL is loaded and injected inside the eye, which is then dialed into the sulcus. Stromal hydration is done and the wound is secured with 10-0 suture if necessary.

PRECAUTIONS

A forceful entry at pars plicata should be avoided during sclerotomy. If resistance is encountered then the chances are that the surgeon is at the level of root of iris. A forceful entry at this juncture can lead to iridodialysis and also hyphema. The trocar or an MVR blade, which is used to create a sclerotomy should be withdrawn and a fresh entry should be attempted slightly below the site of previous entry.

Surgical complications related to the insertion and removal of instruments through the pars plana incisions during vitrectomy have been well described.[1-3] Retinal breaks and dialyses posterior to the sclerotomies are known to occur intraoperatively owing to mechanical traction on the anterior vitreous. A peripheral retinal examination particularly at sclerotomy entry sites before completion of surgery is advocated. Precautions that should be considered include minimizing instrumentation and the number of instrument changes, ensuring good vitreous clearance at sclerotomy sites, and avoiding vitreous incarceration. Multiple uses of disposable instruments, such as the vitrectomy cutter, may be associated with blunting, vitreoretinal traction, and therefore increased occurrence of retinal breaks. Ideally, single-use vitrectomy cutters should not be reused for this reason.

DISCUSSION

This chapter represents and illustrates the surgical approach of pars plicata vitrectomy for phacoemulsification cases complicated by a PCR and residual cortical fragments. Intraoperative PCR is often further precipitated by the constriction of pupil and inability to do a proper vitrectomy as desired by the surgeon.

As pars plicata is further anterior from the vitreous base and Ora serrata, the risk of retinal detachment is lessened. An MVR blade or a trocar cannula can be used to create the sclerotomy incision. The trocar-cannula system has an added advantage of obviating the need for conjunctival incision and providing a self-sealing wound.

The implantation of an acrylic hydrophobic 3-piece foldable IOL in the sulcus and in glued intrascleral IOL fixation preserves the advantages of a small-incision cataract surgery. The modified C-loop haptics of the IOL improves stabilization at the sulcus and applies even, equal tension to the adjacent tissues and the 6.0 mm optic diameter lowers the risk of symptomatic postoperative decentration. Bimanual vitrectomy is preferred in all the cases as a separate infusion prevents the cortical fragments from being pushed away during the chewing up process.

An extensive vitrectomy also prevents pupillary block glaucoma resulting from a vitreous prolapsed into the anterior chamber. Lastly, the vitreous is removed without trauma to the iris, which has been a suspected cause of cystoid macula edema.[4] For anterior segment surgeons who are reluctant to make a pars plana incision following a PCR, this site can be explored and advantage can be availed.

Key Points

- Pars plicata site can be explored for performing anterior vitrectomy.
- It is a safe method and does not carry the risk of damaging the periphery retina or vitreous base.
- It provides very good retro-pupillary access to the rupture site and allows thorough vitrectomy to be done.

REFERENCES

1. Aaberg TM. Pars plana vitrectomy for diabetic tractional retinal detachment. Ophthalmology. 1981;88:639-42.
2. Faulborn J, Conway BP, Machemer R. Surgical complications of pars plana vitreous surgery. Ophthalmology. 1978;85:116-25.
3. Machemer R. A new concept for vitreous surgery: II. Surgical technique and complications. Am J Ophthalmol. 1972;74:1022-33.
4. Grossman SA, Peyman G. Long-term visual results after pars plicata lensectomy-vitrectomy for congenital cataracts. Br J Ophthalmol. 1988; 72:601-6.

Index

Page numbers followed by *t* refer to table and *f* refer to figure